D1396602

The Complete Bicycle Fitness Book

A User's Guide
to the Ultimate
Lifetime Sport
for Exercise, Fun,
and Glowing Health

James C. McCullagh

Editor and Publisher,
Bicycling magazine

WARNER BOOKS 38-234 $8.95 (U.S.A.) 38-235 $10.50 (CAN.)

Rediscover the Joys and Benefits of Cycling!

"The bike has come of age, technologically and aesthetically, and is becoming an essential part of the fitness revolution in America. Used properly and in conjunction with other exercises, cycling can deliver splendid health benefits including: weight loss, lower cholesterol and blood pressure, and reduced resting heart rate. You will read about scores of people of all ages and conditions who have successfully used the bike to help overcome anxiety and depression, as well as debilitating injuries. You will meet people who had difficulty even walking any great distance but who, after a cycling conditioning program, were able to participate in a century, a hundred-mile ride. But to get all these benefits, you will have to know how to ride and use your bicycle. And that is what *The Complete Bicycle Fitness Book* is all about."

—James C. McCullagh,
from the Introduction

The Complete BICYCLE FITNESS Book

James C. McCullagh

Editor and Publisher,
Bicycling magazine

WARNER BOOKS

A Warner Communications Company

Copyright © 1984 by James C. McCullagh

All rights reserved.

Warner Books, Inc., 666 Fifth Avenue, New York, NY 10103

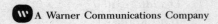 A Warner Communications Company

Printed in the United States of America

First Printing: May 1984

10 9 8 7 6 5 4 3 2

Library of Congress Cataloging in Publication Data

McCullagh, James C.
   The complete bicycle fitness book.

   Bibliography: p. 278
   Includes index.
   1. Cycling. 2. Physical fitness. 3. Cycling—
Physiological aspects. I. Title.
GV1043.7.M33 1984   613.7'1   83-25904
ISBN 0-446-38234-5 (U.S.A.) (pbk.)
        0-446-38235-3 (Canada)

ATTENTION: SCHOOLS AND CORPORATIONS

Warner books are available at quantity discounts with bulk purchase for educational, business, or sales promotional use. For information, please write to: **Special Sales Department, Warner Books, 666 Fifth Avenue, New York, NY 10103.**

ARE THERE WARNER BOOKS YOU WANT
BUT CANNOT FIND IN YOUR LOCAL STORES?

You can get any **Warner Books** title in print. Simply send title and retail price, plus 75¢ per order and 50¢ per copy to cover mailing and handling costs for each book desired. New York State and California residents, add applicable sales tax. Enclose check or money order—no cash, please—to: **Warner Books, PO Box 690, New York, NY 10019. Or send for our complete catalog of Warner Books.**

*For Lee Ann,
Declan, and Dierdre
who know all about
incubation.*

Contents

Acknowledgments

My thanks to the many people in the cycling world who have taught me so much. My thanks to all the racers who have sat patiently through my interviews. My thanks to the *Bicycling* magazine readers who have, directly or indirectly, furthered my education. I am especially grateful to all those cyclists who have shared their personal fitness stories with me. Your fine examples will show the way to many people.

My thanks to Drs. David L. Smith and Eugene A. Gaston, who have been providing solid medical advice to cyclists for more than a decade; to Budd Coates, marathon runner and fitness director at Rodale Press, Inc., for his circuit training routine; to coach Norman Sheil for his weight training tips; to Ed Burke, Ph.D., physiologist and Sports Medicine Director for the United States Cycling Federation, for his guidance; and to the countless writers, researchers and investigators I've had contact with the last eight years.

My special thanks to the *Bicycling* magazine staff from whom I have also learned much, particularly to Senior Editors John Schubert and Tracy DeCrosta for their advice on gearing/training, and nutrition and weight loss, respectively. And to Susan Weaver for her good ideas over the years. I am most grateful.

James C. McCullagh

Introduction

My wife Lee Ann is ecstatic. She stands stiffly in front of me in her red and black cycling clothes and asks me if I notice anything.

"Nothing in particular," I remark, which disappoints her.

"Well, you should," she replies and points delicately to the inside of her thighs.

"Daylight?" I ask. Yes, I had seen the light.

Lee Ann, an enthusiastic cyclist, rope jumper and majorette in her teens, had acquired what were, in her opinion, strong legs. For years she had attempted to slim her legs with all sorts of fitness regimens, from jogging to aerobic dance. They enhanced her general well-being but didn't help her particular problem. As the exercise physiologists put it, those exercises weren't *region-specific*. (If I didn't know better, I'd think they were talking about geography.)

Finally, she had found a way to attack the inside of her thighs: cycling at a brisk cadence. Lee had tried running to reduce the size of her legs. Indeed, before our daughter Deirdre was born, Lee Ann was quite competitive on the running circuit, rarely failing to bring home a medal, ribbon, or a cup. Pleased as she was with her performance, even her 30-to-40-mile weeks didn't reach that pesky part of her legs. But cycling has, and she will ride an easy 25 kilometers (about 16 miles and a one-hour book) to slim her legs. The measuring tape is always handy to help her confront her moment of truth. And if it's telling the truth (she is, of course), Lee Ann has lost a full inch from her legs through a regular (four-to-five-month) cycling program. Given that revelation, she cannot be deterred.

Am I accusing my wife of vanity? Not on your life. I exercise for similar reasons. In the back of my mind is the worthy entreaty from famous cardiologist Dr. Paul Dudley White to start early and exercise for life. But the front of my brain harbors reasons that are more primitive. I expect exercise in general and cycling in particular to contribute to my notion of body image. I want to keep my weight down and my body fat at around ten percent of my total weight.

People buy bikes, people ride bikes, but most Americans have not made the connection between cycling and full body fitness. To be sure, the connection has been made intellectually. Look at some of the old ads from the 1890s, and you will see that a hundred years ago, the bike industry trumpeted the bike as a fitness tool, though, not surprisingly, the medical community warned against the excesses of this new and frivolous sport, particularly for women. Cycling got a real boost when Paul Dudley White, M.D., Eisenhower's physician, stood foursquare behind cycling as an excellent cardiovascular activity, and he certainly influenced the generation of cyclists who took up the sport before the bike boom of 1974.

Dr. White was absolutely right; he was also ahead of his time. Furthermore, his advice was ahead of the quality of equipment being manufactured. Those of you in your forties will likely remember the heavy-duty "newsboy" bikes popular in the late fifties and sixties. These steel-framed bikes were reliable to a fault, but they were a far cry from the lightweight, multigeared, dependable ten-speeds we have today. Thus, when Dr. White was encouraging Americans to climb aboard bikes, the equipment really wasn't there, at least not for the population at large.

And the difference between the concept of fitness today and what existed twenty years ago is significant. In the early sixties fitness in America meant doing a certain number of push-ups, sit-ups, and pull-ups within a prescribed time limit. John F. Kennedy's New Frontier brought some changes in that perception but not much.

Today's bikes might look the same as those sold ten years ago, but much has really changed. The technology has improved so that there is a wide selection of lightweight, dependable, multispeed bikes that will deliver maximum fitness benefits. The bike has come of age, technologically and aesthetically, and is becoming an essential part of the fitness revolution in America. Used properly and in conjunction with other exercises, cycling can deliver splendid health benefits including: weight loss, lower cholesterol and blood pressure, and reduced resting heart rate.

You will read about scores of people of all ages and conditions who have successfully used the bike to help overcome anxiety and depression, as well as debilitating injuries. You will meet people who had difficulty even *walking* any great distance but who, after a cycling conditioning program, were able to participate in a *century*—a hundred-mile ride.

But to get all these benefits, you will have to know how to ride and use your bicycle. And that is what *The Complete Bicycle Fitness Book* is all about. It will show you how to get started, improve your technique, participate in a variety of training programs. It will show you how to make the bicycle a central part of your fitness schedule and how to balance and complement your cycling with related activities such as running and cross-country skiing. A lengthy chapter is devoted to total body fitness, including various options for indoor cycling and weight training.

This book will show you what to eat and consume for maximum energy. It provides a complete weight-loss program and an introduction to new electronic and computer tools that will help you monitor your fitness level.

In short, you will learn everything you need to know to build a complete fitness program around cycling.

The Complete Bicycle Fitness Book will concentrate on the use of the bike—not the bike itself. I have included enough information on equipment choices to get you started, but *you* are the main character, not the bicycle.

Cycling is an equal opportunity fitness activity, ideally suited to both men and women. I embrace that notion and, except where physiology dictates specific advice for either men or women, offer all recommendations in that spirit.

In organization, this book is developmental, though you can certainly jump ahead to later chapters, depending on your present level of fitness. By following the recommendations in this book, you will certainly get fitter. You might even transform your life.

1

Lifesport

I travel a lot and on my journeys I'm bombarded with how-to tips on keeping fit, from moving my toes in flight to mimicking the armchair antics of a model who leads me through the motions over a hotel's closed-circuit television system. The advice is offered in the proper spirit, and I always learn something in the process. I'm convinced, however, that if exercise becomes another form of tedium, homogenized and completely separated from the principle of pleasure and enjoyment, then it won't contribute significantly to our long-term fitness.

Frequently in this book you will see the word *lifesport* referring to activities a person can participate in for a lifetime as opposed to those more traditional competitive sports that suit us only in our earlier, most strenuously active years.

Daily we are introduced to instant diets and other gimmicks that will trim our waists and melt off unwanted fat. Unfortunately, we know that there are few secret or instant regimens. There is no magic routine. We should acknowledge early on that fitness is a *lifetime* pursuit. And in that case, why not make it as pleasant and rewarding as possible? Why not choose an activity you can stay with, one that offers endless variety, one that is kind to your mind and body?

You might think that *lifesport* has an ominous ring. Do you mean that I will have to do *something* for the rest of my life if I'm going to be fit? Yes, that's exactly right. But take heart, you won't have to be a triathlete or a superstar. Research has shown that you can readily get by on very little exercise. Furthermore, you are never too old to get started. Above all, the emphasis should be on *frequency* not *intensity* of exercise.

Researchers for the Netherlands Heart Foundation have shown that very gentle activities such as walking, cycling or gardening *without seasonal interruption* lessen the risk of heart attack (*American Journal of Epidemiology*, 1979). Similar studies have shown that people who walk or cycle to work each morning are less likely to have heart problems than people who do little more than engage in summer gardening activities.

In other words, sustained, light physical activity lessens the risk of heart attack. And the emphasis should be on *sustained*. Killing yourself for the summer or on an occasional weekend will not do you any good. Furthermore, we know that if you stop exercising completely, within 10 to 14 days you'll begin to lose the fitness benefits you've gained.

Keep in mind that if you want to reach a minimal fitness level, you really don't have to devote that much time a week to exercise. Kenneth H. Cooper, M.D., who made *aerobic* a household word, has recently recommended to the White House Symposium on Physical Fitness and Sports Medicine that you don't gain that much from running more than 15 miles a week, which will satisfy most of the conditions of a cardiovascular conditioning program. Researchers at the Norwegian Health Sport Center found that ten minutes of exercise a day is enough to improve the ability of your lungs to handle oxygen, though the study suggests you would have to exercise at least 30 minutes, three times a week to significantly improve cardiovascular function and positively influence factors associated with the aging process (*Scandinavian Journal of Social Medicine*, 1982).

Surveys that ask why people exercise usually find weight loss and improved body image at the top of the list. I suspect a primary reason people exercise is to slow the aging process. We all want to be able to be as active in our 60s and 70s as we are or were in our 20s and 30s.

Research has yet to prove that exercise will enable us to live longer. Yet according to the President's Council on Physical Fitness and Sports, people could avoid many of the infirmities associated with old age if they were more active. In simple terms exercise makes us breathe oxygen and oxygen feeds and rejuvenates our body cells. So when you exercise your heart and lungs, your entire body benefits. And it's never too late to start.

It used to be thought that our ability to train diminishes with age, that people over 60 could benefit little from a training program. That is no longer believed. In fact, researchers have shown that older people react to training in almost the same way as the young, though it might take a longer period to gain the same training effect.

While it is never too late to start an exercise program, the benefits of staying with one for a lifetime are apparent. A group of lifelong British cyclists over 50 was examined to determine just what a lifetime of cycling would contribute to the overall health of the heart. This group, members of the Fellowship of Cycling Old Timers, had cycled 5,000 to 10,000 miles a year when they were younger and 2,000 miles more recently. Seventy-five percent of the 300 questioned still cycled regularly throughout the year. Fifty-four of the over-70 group cycled once a week or more throughout the year. Compared with the general population, this group had fewer heart attacks and heart problems.

And the over-75 group had a tenfold decrease in the incidence of all heart disease (*British Medical Journal*, December, 1977).

There seems little doubt that regular cycling contributed to the state of health in the Fellowship of Cycling Old Timers. I don't think it was any accident that the average age of death for these cyclists was 79, far above the British and American average.

So there is every reason to believe that both men and women can maintain a high level of fitness well into their 70s and 80s. And as you have seen, cycling is a splendid and appropriate lifesport which can help protect the heart, improve the capacity of the lungs, and keep your body lean.

The beauty of the bike is that the machine is quite adaptable to the requirements of our age and ability. Nowhere is this adaptability clearer than in the use of bicycle gearing, the great equalizer. I'll be discussing the subject in some detail in Chapter Six, but let me say here that the multispeed gearing on modern, lightweight bikes is not only beneficial to the beginner who wants to ease into the sport but also to the older cyclist who can't travel as fast as a 20-year-old.

Here is a chart prepared by Eugene A. Gaston, M.D., a doctor and a cyclist. Dr. Gaston shows how, for a 25-mile time trial on a flat coarse with no wind, horsepower decreases significantly between ages 20 and 70. However, there is not such a pronounced drop in speed (miles per hour) and time. His conclusion:

> Cycling is an ideal lifetime exercise for both athlete and nonathlete. Even those with relatively low power outputs will make good time on the level terrain, and thanks to modern day, wide-range gearing with gears descending into the low 20s, the reasonably fit septua-

genarian can climb steep grades without straining or
getting off and walking.

TABLE ONE

Age	Horsepower Output	Speed (mph)	Time for 25 miles (hours: minutes) (rounded to nearest ½ minute)
20	0.45	25	1:0
30	0.40	24	1:2.5
35	0.38	23.6	1:3.5
40	0.36	23.2	1:4.5
45	0.34	22.8	1:6
50	0.32	22.4	1:7
55	0.306	22.1	1:8
60	0.29	21.8	1:9
65	0.28	21.6	1:9.5
70	0.27	21.4	1:10

According to Shinichi Toriyama, a bicycle physiologist,
cycling contributes to health because it upgrades the
function of the circulatory system, upgrades the function
of the respiratory system, and provides easy access to
exercise requiring high oxygen consumption (*JBPI* Bulletin).

In a strictly nonmedical, nontechnical sense, I like to
think of the leg muscles as kind of a second heart. The
largest muscles in the body are concentrated in the lower
limbs and are powerfully involved through the act of
pedaling. The pedaling process, simply put, helps the
heart, supplying large quantities of blood for each contraction.
Toriyama notes that "because of the smoother flow of
blood, vessels become more flexible and undesirable deposits
on the inner walls are more readily eliminated. As

the blood carries a large amount of energy source material (in the form of glucose in the blood vessels) and oxygen, new blood is continuously produced and the number of red blood cells is increased. Cholesterol is reduced."

During the act of pedaling the muscles use large amounts of stored muscle fuel and oxygen and transport wastes and carbon dioxide to be excreted. New capillary vessels are formed. Because cycling can be done for long periods of time without ill effects, it results in a large consumption of oxygen. And the consumption of oxygen is a factor in the utilization of body fat.

The accompanying chart represents a modification of the physiological benefits of cycling as outlined by Toriyama. The benefits read like a prescription for good health. Through energetic—not casual—cycling, you can expand the capacity of your heart, decrease your resting pulse, increase your training pulse, increase oxygen uptake, reduce cholesterol, enhance circulation, improve blood flow and more. In other words, regular cycling can deliver all the benefits usually associated with *full-body fitness*, a notion that receives support from medical authorities around the world.

The long-term, exhaustive Farmington Heart Study has important implications for the fitness-minded cyclist. One important medical finding of the Farmington Heart Study Group, as reported in *Bicycling* magazine by Dr. Gaston, suggests that cycling as little as 25 miles a week can reduce your risk of coronary heart disease. Specifically, the study showed that recreational cyclists seem to have the *right* amount of the *right* kind of cholesterol.

It is common knowledge that coronary heart disease is epidemic in this country, affecting 1 in 5 men over 60 and 1 in every 17 women. The disease is caused by obstructions in the coronary arteries which result from a buildup of cholesterol. What makes us prone: obesity,

TABLE TWO
PHYSIOLOGICAL BENEFITS OF CYCLING

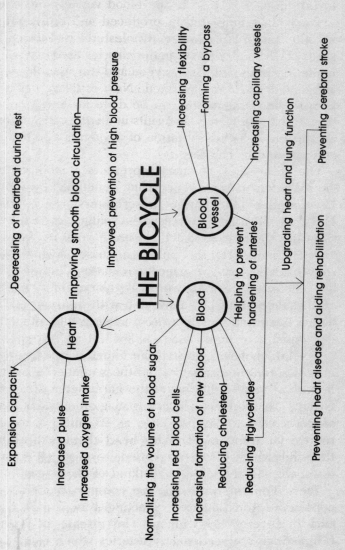

THE BICYCLE

Heart
- Expansion capacity
- Increased pulse
- Increased oxygen intake
- Decreasing of heartbeat during rest
- Improving smooth blood circulation
- Improved prevention of high blood pressure

Blood vessel
- Increasing flexibility
- Forming a bypass
- Increasing capillary vessels
- Helping to prevent hardening of arteries

Blood
- Normalizing the volume of blood sugar
- Increasing red blood cells
- Increasing formation of new blood
- Reducing cholesterol
- Reducing triglycerides

- Upgrading heart and lung function
- Preventing cerebral stroke
- Preventing heart disease and aiding rehabilitation

cigarette smoking, lack of exercise and blood cholesterol levels.

Dr. Gaston notes that new discoveries indicate that it's not the amount of cholesterol that is important but the kind. HDL (high density lipoprotein) cholesterol prevents hardening of the arteries and may even reverse the process. HDL cholesterol is "good" cholesterol. LDL, low density lipoprotein, is hence the "bad" cholesterol, the kind that clogs up the arteries, and can be attributed in part to a diet heavy in saturated fats.

According to Dr. Gaston,

> What is new and exciting about cholesterol is the proof, by the Farmington Heart Study and others, that the total amount in the blood is less important than the ratio of total cholesterol to HDL cholesterol. The more HDL in the total cholesterol, the lower the incidence of coronary disease. The amount of HDL cholesterol can be increased by exercise, but if the total cholesterol is simultaneously reduced, the ratio is even better. The ratio is calculated by dividing the amount of total blood cholesterol by the amount of HDL cholesterol; the lower the ratio, the less the risk of coronary disease.

Table Three shows a man with a total cholesterol count of 350 and an HDL of 70. The ratio is 5, and this represents an average risk for men. Note what happens when he changes the ratio. Either lowering total cholesterol or raising HDL cholesterol will reduce the risk.

Table Four shows ratios for various segments of the population. And Table Five provides information about the Charles River Wheelmen who participated in the study. Interestingly, recreational cyclists had a risk factor similar to marathon runners, who presumably devote more time to their training.

TABLE THREE

Total Cholesterol HDL Cholesterol	Ratio	Risk of Developing Coronary Heart Disease (CHD)
350 (mg per 100 ml) / 70	5	Standard risk for men
250 / 70	3.4	Half the standard risk
300 / 88.2	3.4	Half the standard risk

TABLE FOUR

RATIOS OF TOTAL TO HDL CHOLESTEROL FRAMINGHAM HEART STUDY

	RATIO OF TOTAL CHOLESTEROL HDL CHOLESTEROL
Vegetarians	2.8
One-half standard risk	3.4
Boston Marathon runners	3.4
Standard risk (women)	4.4
Standard risk (men)	5.0
Average CHD victim (male)	5.4
Twice standard risk (women)	7.1
(men)	9.6
Three times standard risk (women)	11.0
(men)	23.4

TABLE FIVE
CHARLES RIVER WHEELMEN

	Women	Men	Total
Number of riders	6	10	16
Average ages	40.5	45.5	43.5
Average bicycle miles per week	25	108	77
Additional participation in other sports (hrs/wk)	7	10	9
Total cholesterol HDL cholesterol	3.0	3.9	3.6

What can be done to develop and maintain a low total/HDL ratio? Here's what Dr. Gaston advises:
• Exercise regularly. Endurance exercise, such as bicycling, running, swimming, or cross-country skiing, is best.
• Do not smoke.
• Maintain—and if necessary, regain—your ideal weight. For most people this is the weight at young maturity, between the ages of 21 and 23.
• Limit the intake of saturated fat and cholesterol; substitute polyunsaturated fat.
—Eliminate butter fat. Use skimmed milk, margarine and low-fat (one percent) or nonfat cottage cheese.
—Eat less beef, lamb and pork. Remove the fat. Avoid gravy.
—Avoid the skin of poultry. It contains most of the fat.
—Eat more fish. Fish fat is polyunsaturated.
—Use polyunsaturated oil (safflower oil is best) for salads and cooking.
—Egg yolks are nearly 100 percent cholesterol, and liver contains large amounts. Avoid both. Egg whites are pure, high-grade protein and excellent nutrition.

•   Alcohol, in moderation, favorably affects the total/HDL ratio.

If cycling can help ward off coronary heart disease, it can also help bring back to full and active lives those who have suffered heart attacks. That fact has been established and proven by a Specialized Coronary Outpatient Rehabilitation (SCOR) program in California, developed to assist middle-aged men who have coronary arteriosclerosis (hardening of the arteries). Clinically speaking, this is a disease of the arteries which restricts the flow of blood to the heart muscle, resulting in heart attack or angina (chest pain).

According to Randy Ice, the physical therapist who organized the program, there are thirty patients in the group, "all of whom have had either a heart attack, angina pectoris, or coronary bypass surgery." Under carefully supervised medical conditions, Ice led SCOR patients on gentle rides over very flat terrain but only after they had participated in a hospital-based exercise program for two or three months.

The first ride was 24 miles, covered in more than three hours. That was the first of a number of remarkable achievements. Eleven years later, most patients have participated in a century ride (100 miles) with some riding double centuries. A crowning achievement was the SCOR cross-country relay ride completed in 12 days by 14 participants ranging in age from 47 to 66 (I have ridden with some of these cyclists and can attest to what shape they are in).

During the course of the program, three patients suffered repeat heart attacks, though these incidences seemed to be associated with continued cigarette smoking. Overall, the SCOR cyclists have performed remarkably and are now well on their way to logging 500,000 miles, which encourages Ice to remark that "long-distance bicycling is a safe method of improving the exercise capacity of the patient with coronary heart disease and is conducive to the type of life-style which enhances the heart patient's chance of survival."

Examples of individuals who have used cycling to come back from heart attacks abound, both inside and outside of the published medical literature. W. E. Mattey of Bristol, West Virginia, had a heart attack when he was 67 and spent nine days in the intensive care unit. On the advice of his doctor he started a modest cycling program. At first he was unable to cycle more than a quarter of a mile. A year later he did his first century. Now he has logged over 20,000 miles and is still going strong. His doctor says if it weren't for cycling he probably wouldn't have survived.

Although I'm a firm believer in medical studies and hope the current interest in cycling and fitness will encourage more researchers to look at the long-term benefits of cycling, I put considerable stock in my personal and anecdotal experiences.

"Know thyself" is among the oldest and best advice. With proper instruction there is no reason that you cannot monitor your own body, cannot take your own pulse and blood pressure. (I'll talk about keeping a diary and a record of your training later in this book.) For example, when my resting pulse gets above 60, which I consider too high, it is usually because I am stressed. By taking my pulse regularly, I know how to respond, usually through exercise or some kind of stress control, such as meditation. Part of the appeal and responsibility of full-body fitness is to be able to monitor yourself and your training. "Know thyself."

To get a better sense of how beginning cyclists keep track of their own fitness, I surveyed 500 people who participated in a cycling training program at the Lehigh County Velodrome (racing track) near Allentown, Pennsylvania. The riders got their start on the velodrome but did most riding on the road.

The average age of the respondents was 31; nearly 90 percent were men. Of the respondents, 84 percent indicated that their level of fitness had improved and nearly half had lost weight. Most of the riders who wanted to lose weight did. Lost weight ranged from 5 to 75 pounds, with the average being nearly 20 pounds.

As these findings indicate, once you make cycling a part of your life, you accrue many benefits. Your weight will likely drop or stabilize, your resting pulse will probably go down. You will certainly become more conscious of your body, of what you eat and what you do. Interestingly, many people start cycling just for the fun of it and reap enormous benefits nonetheless. Roger McGill of Sellersville, Pennsylvania, lost 75 pounds in one year. His resting pulse dropped from 70 to 55. And he now enjoys additional energy and pep.

As a fitness tool and activity, cycling knows no bounds. No matter what your present level of fitness, you can start cycling on your own terms and progress at your own rate.

2

Getting Started

I t is not uncommon for adults, feeling the weight of too many pounds, to jump on the first bike handy. That means that many recreational cyclists—and I venture to say the majority— are cycling on ill-fitting bikes. It could be that the frame is too small, the seat too low, or the stem too long.

Fit. *Cardinal Rule Number One:* You'll make it easier on yourself and will make your cycling more fun and rewarding if you ride a bike that fits.

So where do you begin? Chances are you already have a bike. If so, you should check whether it fits properly. You might have been sold a bike by a salesperson who asked you to straddle a bike. If there's an inch or half-inch clearance between your crotch and the top tube, the bike fits you. Right?

Probably—though as you will see, there are a number of other considerations. The above description presents a reasonable rule of thumb and a place to start. If women are not uncomfortable on a bike with a top tube, I would recommend riding one; it is more responsive and flexes less than a traditional woman's frame, called a *mixte*. But you will discover in the next chapter there's more to bike fit than straddling the top tube. After all, we come in all shapes and sizes. If you are to use your existing bike as a fitness tool, it should fit you like a glove. You won't stay with cycling long if you develop back, wrist and neck pains from a badly fitting bike.

Consumers often spend more time trying on a pair of shoes than trying on a bike. Furthermore, the act of fitting the bike to your frame is complicated, because while frame sizes—which refer to the length of the seat tube—are usually standardized and come in 19-, 21-, 23-, and 25-inch lengths, the length of some of the component parts is variable. For example, you could buy a 19-inch frame with a 19¾-inch or 21¼-inch top tube, the length of the imaginary line that intersects the seat tube and the head tube. While the inch-and-a-half difference in top tube length might not seem much on paper, it would if you had short arms and torso, *which happens to be how many women are built*. You would have to stretch out to reach the handlebars, even if you were riding on the "tops." If you were riding on the "drops," you would be stretched out even more.

Advice. Spend a great deal of time fitting the bike to you, not because it is complicated, but because your cycling will be much more pleasurable and efficient. Women should be particularly inquisitive and demanding because by and large the bikes currently on the market have been designed to men's proportions. Men are typically longer in the torso and have shorter legs; women typically have a proportionately shorter torso and a longer inseam. If you have to reach too far for the handlebars, the bike doesn't fit you. While with exercise and stretching, you will become more supple and will be able to reach the handlebar drops with little difficulty, you will not grow into an ill-fitting bike.

While you are sitting on a bike, or, better still, road-testing it, be aware of your ability to reach the brakes, whether operated from the top or bottom of the handlebars. Make sure that the distance between the handlebar drop and the brake lever—the *reach*—is not too far for your own reach.

Gearing. We'll get into gearing in detail in a later chapter. If you are shopping for a bike you should know that most bikes sold over the counter have gearing that is not designed for the beginner cyclist; that is, at one end of the range it is too high, and at the other end, not low enough. Before you actually put your money down, you should glance at Chapter Six. Ask the salesperson a straightforward question about the range of gearing measured in inches and whether the range on the bike in question is appropriate for your kind of riding. I'd recommend a low of around 30 inches and a high gear of 90 inches. If the gearing on the bike is not appropriate, the shop can make a minor adjustment, such as changing a cog on the rear wheel, so you get the gearing most appropriate for you. And don't think of this as technical mumbo jumbo. The right gearing on a bike will make your cycling a real pleasure. Have you ever noticed the many people pushing their bikes up hills? Some of them look very strong and fit. I've made it a point to stop and talk to these people from time to time. On almost every occasion the culprit is too high a gearing. Manufacturers are slowly coming around to the notion that you don't cycle to acquire big leg muscles but rather to improve your cardiovascular system.

The first question many newcomers to the sport ask is: How many speeds should I buy—which suggests if you buy more speeds (gears), you will somehow go faster. And for some reason there has been a cultural bias which says women need fewer gears than men. When I purchased my first bike as an adult some 15 years ago, the Schwinn shop owner immediately steered me to a five speed and my wife to a three. The result was that Lee Ann really had to strain going up hills.

Don't think of gears in terms of speeds. Gears provide a mechanical advantage that enables you to pedal at an optimum rate no matter how steep the terrain is. Having more gears on a bike won't necessarily mean you will go faster; they mean you will, if you use them properly, be a more accomplished and efficient cyclist.

So how many speeds do you need? If you are going to use your bicycle primarily as a fitness tool, get yourself a 10-speed, which I use generically. Many bikes these days are actually 12- and 18-speeds. If the gearing is intelligently designed, these bikes are a pleasure to ride.

Where to Look.   If you don't have a bike or are thinking about trading your old one in, where should you go? Generally speaking, you can buy bikes in mass merchandisers, such as Sears, and specialty bike shops. Since you are going to use your bike as a fitness tool, you are probably better off buying from a specialty shop simply because you will get professional help regarding bike fit. Bike shops have experienced people who can properly set up a bike to match your physical makeup and riding style.

Cost.   The median price of a bike sold through U.S. specialty shops is around $215. In other words, half the bikes sold are below that price, half above. What should you spend? I would recommend that you invest at least that median figure. Contrary to popular notion, bikes are very good investments and the product category experiencing the least inflation in the last five years. And keep in mind that a good bike at the turn of the century would have cost you $50 to $60.

Brand.   What brand of bicycle should you buy? Over the years I've been involved in road-testing nearly a thousand bikes and in recent years I've found few I couldn't recommend. The bicycle has been around for a hundred years and for most of its life has been a mass-produced item. Thus procedures and technologies to produce the basic frame tubing have been perfected. In our laboratory tests we've found that some tubing is stronger than others under extreme stress, but for the recreational cyclists that measure has no particular meaning.

There is intense competition in the bicycle marketplace, particularly between domestic and foreign manufacturers, a struggle that doesn't have any clear parameters because many of the bikes sold by domestic manufacturers are made in Taiwan and Japan. A legitimate but not particularly revealing question—given the standardization of manufacturing processes—is where a bike is made.

The fact is the bike that waits for you in American shops is an international bike which might have frame tubing from Britain, components from Italy, and rims from Japan. And the brands are almost too numerous to mention. They include: Schwinn, Ross, Murray, Huffy, Trek, Fuji, Bridgestone, Miyata, Panasonic, Centurion, Bianchi, Lotus, Takara, Raleigh, Univega, Peugot, Motobecane, Gitan and many more.

The fact that there are so many brands and so much competition is good news for the consumer. The competition has kept the prices down and given you a much better choice. And keep in mind that where you buy your bike is as important as what you buy.

Weight. The automobile buyer who kicks the tires of a prospective purchase has become a part of American lore. So has the consumer who picks up the bike before he puts his money down. It is certainly a natural inclination to see how much the bike weighs, but you should know that where the weight is found on a bike is more important than the total weight. Most $200-plus bikes weigh 30 pounds or less, so overall weight is generally not a problem. What you want to be concerned about is whether the bike's drivetrain (rims, pedals, cranks and chainwheels) is made of steel or an alloy. If these parts are made of steel, you will feel the weight much more than if it's in the frame. The bike will feel heavier and less responsive and you are much less likely to use it as an exercise tool.

Handlebars The multispeed bike I'm referring to will have dropped or "racing" handlebars, the advantage being that you can put your hand in a number of distinct positions, depending on the type of riding you are doing. You might, because of preference or physical condition, want a bike with upright handlebars. If so, tell the salesperson. For those who like riding in the upright position and appreciate the wider saddles, you might consider a new category of bikes called all-terrain bikes that offer all the advantages of a lightweight, multispeed bike but with a wider saddle and tires and upright handlebars. However, due to the upright design of the bike, you are not likely to get as good a workout on this model as on a traditional ten-speed.

Toe Clips. The salesperson is likely to have asked you about toe clips, the metal cage and leather straps that help keep your feet secure on the pedals. Because toe clips contribute so much to your riding efficiency, you should purchase them, which are frequently standard equipment on bikes over $200. Depending on your riding experience, you might choose not to use them until you become more comfortable on the bike. But make sure you have them.

If you're shopping for a bike, get a multispeed bike with alloy wheels and drivetrain components (referred to above). Figure on spending at least $215. And buy from a store that lets you road-test the bike. *Spend what you need to spend to get these features*.

In suggesting a price of $215 I'm talking about a suitable bike for an entry level cyclist who wants to make the bike a central part of his or her fitness program. You can, of course, pay more for a bike. More expensive bikes offer more in the way of better machine parts and generally a more satisfactory riding experience. You'll pay more for the top-of-the-line Campagnola, Shimano or Suntour derailleurs that are crisp and smooth shifting, a pleasure to use. You will pay more for lightweight and sturdy Reynolds or Columbus tubing and will feel the difference beneath you. If you want to hear the "sing" of exotic Clement tires—called "silks"—you will pay for that level of ecstasy. And, in time, you might consider it worth it. You might even consider buying a custom bike, especially made for you, which will certainly add to your cycling enjoyment. But for now, you can get fit for less. As I talk about "getting better" and getting more out of your exercise program, I'll suggest ways you can upgrade your bike.

Bikes that cost around $215 have features you might or might not prefer. Consumer preference at this price level dictates that most of the bikes have "auxiliary" brake levers, a kind of secondary brake that allows you to operate it while your hands are resting on the top of the handlebars. Surveys have shown that most beginners like these levers, perhaps because they seem to provide an added measure of protection.

If you feel more comfortable with them on a bike, that's fine. You should know that with these auxiliary levers you lose some mechanical advantage, particularly if the levers are not adjusted properly, which is often the case. If you think you can get by without them, ask the salesperson to remove them.

To the aficionado, where the gear shift levers appear on a bike is an item of great importance. Few enthusiasts would ride a bike if the shifts were on the handlebars rather than the downtube. Why? Simply because the closer the actual gear shift levers are to the front and rear derailleurs, the better, more crisp the shifting. While that is absolutely true, you might feel a little uncomfortable at first reaching down between your legs to shift gears. *Advice:* Go with whatever is comfortable for you. In time you will be able to brake, shift gears, watch for traffic and probably take a drink from your water bottle, all while keeping your bike well under control. If a component or feature will make your cycling more enjoyable, then use it. There is no virtue in having a bike with all the recommended features and not using it.

A Rule of Thumb: Buy the lowest-priced 10- (or 12-) speed bicycle with aluminum wheels from a full-time maker and a bicycle shop you can trust.

What to Wear. While I will be discussing "Dressing for Fitness" in detail later on (Chapter Nine), a few quick words here will be helpful.

You know you can ride a bike in any kind of clothes and you can likely get fit in the process. Cycling clothing is very functional. Cycling shorts, with a partial chamois lining, help reduce the irritation caused by the movement of the buttocks on the saddle. When you cycle for exercise and fitness, you will be cycling at more than 80 revolutions per minute and if you are wearing shorts and cutoffs, you will irritate your skin. So there are good physiological reasons for investing $25 in cycling shorts.

Most people cycle in T-shirts and tanktops, which is quite appropriate if they are cycling around the block, unless they run the risk of sunburn. But if you're cycling for fitness, at different speeds in different weather where you experience rapid changes in temperature, you should wear a cycling jersey that helps "wick off" your perspiration and reduce the wind chill.

Shoes. If you want to pedal at a brisk pace for fitness,

sooner or later you will have to make an investment in cycling shoes. Most of us have had the experience of pedaling in street shoes and having our feet slip off the pedal when we crank it up. The shinbone usually receives the blow.

Helmets. Cycling is a safe activity and particularly safe in the hands of experienced practitioners. Yes, cyclists get hurt and killed but these are usually children or inexperienced cyclists. However, cyclists live in the real world and on roads populated by cars, and prudence demands that you protect your head with a hard shell helmet, if only as a precautionary measure. Your bike shop has a good supply of helmets in your size. *Buy one and wear it.*

If you started out from scratch and had to purchase a bike and choose to purchase the other items I mentioned, you've probably spent around $350, a pretty reasonable cost to get you in shape for life.

Finally, if you haven't been on a bike for years, you should find a quiet spot such as a parking lot and get used to the feel of the machine. Practice shifting the gears under light pedal pressure. Learn which shifter, located on the handlebars or down tube, controls the front or rear derailleur. Look down and witness the chain move (be "derailled") from one chainwheel or cog to the others. Practice squeezing the brake, gently. Note which brake controls which wheel.

3

Relaxing on a Bike

I recall visiting the training camp of Japanese professional cyclists. These young men, aged 18 to 24, are brought to a quiet training camp in the mountains where they can learn the lucrative trade of Keirin (track) racing. Some of these men have had cycling experience, some have not. The coaches separate the two categories and instruct the novices for months on very basic cycling maneuvers, such as turns and figure-eights. These tough, strong men are not permitted with the other cyclists until they know how to handle their bikes.

Now let's come closer to home.

During the ABC telecast of the 1981 Iron Man Triathlon in Hawaii, a commentator remarked about the fluid movements of veteran cyclist John Howard, the eventual winner. The speaker couldn't get over Howard's ability to cycle almost effortlessly, riding no hands while he enjoyed a drink from his water bottle. That day, Howard was a study in proper bike position and fit. Howard didn't fight with the handlebars or grip them tightly, a failing of many new cyclists; he "laid" on them with his hands, letting his powerful leg muscles do the work. Howard didn't stay glued to the handlebar drops; he moved his hands around the bars, looking for a comfortable position and rest for his body.

Howard's ability to relax on a bike while still turning a big gear in a high pedal cadence was the result of tens of thousands of miles of training and racing, spanning more than a decade. And while you are unlikely to ever generate Howard's power, you can learn how to relax on your bike, letting as much energy as possible be translated into turning the wheels.

In a nutshell: Position on a bike is everything. Over time, proper position on a bike feels better. It allows you to relax, so you can spend hours in the saddle without undue aches and soreness. Without proper position, you'll ride tentatively, and you'll hurt more.

Good position has to be acquired, like a taste for some wines or strong coffee. It doesn't feel natural at first—but neither does a good golf swing or ski position. It's after you've worked at it awhile that it brings its benefits to your cycling—and at that point you'll never want to go back to any of the aspects of poor position.

Let's go around the bike and make adjustments everywhere there's an adjustment to be made.

Saddle Height.   Saddle height is the single most important aspect of position; get this right and the rest will follow. It's easy to get it right, but a high percentage of cyclists get it wrong.

Many novice cyclists want to start out with their saddles very low, so they can touch the ground with both their feet while remaining in the saddle, a practice that goes back to the days of the bicycle hobbyhorse (1870) which one propelled with his feet. This might seem like fun and you might think it a safe practice but it isn't.

With your saddle low, your legs will be bent too much, which means that you won't be getting maximum benefits from your "second heart." You won't be able to spin the pedals in any meaningful cadence and therefore won't push oxygen-laden blood through your system. But you will wear out your shoes.

When a cyclist gains a little more confidence in his ability to handle the bike, he may want to raise the saddle much higher, so the leg is fully extended at the bottom of the pedal stroke. This too is a mistake. It feels good to a novice cyclist, because it uses the same muscles in the same way that walking does. But cycling isn't walking, and an in-between position will help you cycle better.

Many cyclists are skeptical of this. The saddle feels good when it's too high; why should they lower it and feel more cramped? The answer is: Try it for a couple weeks and see the results.

A good rule of thumb, recommended by the National Cycling Coach, followed by many top competitive cyclists and coaches, is that your saddle should be at a height such that when you put your *heels* on the pedals (assuming you use toe clips, this means you use the underside of the pedals to conduct this test) you can pedal freely without having to rock your buttocks from side to side to reach the bottom of the pedal stroke. Have a friend hold the bike upright while you sit on it, and backpedal to perform this test.

Now, when you put the ball of your foot on the pedal, which is the foot position you should always use when you ride, your knee will always be slightly bent at the bottom of each pedal stroke.

Why not have your saddle higher, so you can stretch your leg out straight with each stroke? The biggest reason is that you can spin better with your saddle lower. If your saddle is too low, you cannot engage your quadricep muscles to their fullest. For years, I rode with my saddle about two inches too high. Try as I did to develop a good spin, my sprint spin never got above 110 rpm, and my cruising cadence was about 30 rpm below that. Within a year after lowering my saddle, I increased my springing cadence to 160, and I felt *comfortable* spinning at 100 to 110 when the occasion demanded it.

The benefit of a good spin will be fully explained in later sections on cadence and gearing, but the benefits of a lower saddle don't end with a brisk cadence. It's easier to stay smooth on the bike when you have the saddle low enough. If you have the opportunity to watch top bike riders in your area—perhaps at a race sponsored by your local club—notice their form. Their legs may churn like eggbeaters while their upper bodies remain motionless. In fact, some racing cyclists emphasize this point by riding a stationary exercise bike while balancing books atop their heads.

Staying smooth allows you to steer the bike better—the bike doesn't wobble down the road, veering left as you lunge at the right pedal, and vice versa. It allows you to control the bike's position on the pavement well, so you can use the bike's position to give an exact signal of your intentions to other road users (along with the appropriate hand signals). Your steadiness on the bike is a welcome signal to other road users that you are truly in control of your vehicle.

Physiologists and coaches at the United States Cycling Federation Training Center in Colorado Springs devised a test to determine optimum saddle height. Cyclists pedaled a bike with a hydraulic seat post that could be raised and lowered at will. However, the formula that was developed from these tests didn't work for everyone. For example, some women couldn't reach the pedals at the so-called ideal saddle height. So much for formula.

Another formula that has been kicked around the cycling world suggests your saddle height—from floor to saddle— should be anywhere from 105 to 109 percent of your inseam measurement. This measurement is taken while

you are standing without shoes and represents a reasonable rule of thumb for the fitness-minded recreational
cyclist, though chances are the preceding advice will
likely put you in the middle of the above percentage.

Keep in mind that these are not unimportant measurements. When Greg LeMond, America's best professional
road racer, went to ride for the Renault team in France,
one of the first things Renault did was to run wind tunnel
tests on LeMond to determine his best riding position.
The tests indicated that he would be more efficient and
ride more aerodynamically if his seat were about two
centimeters higher. And this small change helped improve
his cycling. He was stronger and could climb better. For a
professional, being able to ride more comfortably and
efficiently during a 160-mile stage race is crucial, particularly in light of the fact that many of these races are won
by seconds—not minutes.

Whether you are riding one mile or one hundred,
correct saddle height is as important for you as for the best
professional riders. You are worth the fuss—so are your
knees.

Foot Position and Toe Clip Placement. As stated
above, the ball of your foot should be atop the pedal. You
can place your foot more precisely than that too: Your foot
should be in the exact position which places the ball
directly atop the pedal spindle.

If you're used to pedaling with your arch on the pedal,
this too may feel unfamiliar. Even if you have too-long toe
clips, they may feel right, since they will place the ball of
your foot as much as an inch ahead of the pedal spindle.

These small errors in position make for a big penalty in
performance: They keep four of the most powerful muscles in your body from helping you propel the bike! Each
leg has two calf muscles available to help you point your

toes downward and move the pedal through its range of
motion. The muscles can't do their job, though, if your
foot is too far forward on the pedals.

It's unlikely that you have your feet too far back on the
pedals, with the ball of the foot behind the crank spindle.
This foot position feels more unnatural than having your
foot too far forward, so people generally avoid it.

If you don't use toe clips, you'll find that it takes some
concentration to hold your foot in the proper position on
the pedals, particularly as you reach for the higher cadences that are the subject of the next chapter.

For this reason, most other cycling books on the market
will tell you dogmatically that you must use toe clips. But
today there's a very legitimate place for the bicycle *enthusiast*
(remember, not every bicycle user is an enthusiast) who
doesn't use toe clips.

That place is on the lightweight fat-tire bikes designed
for off-road use called all-terrain bikes. If you ride one of
these on rough dirt trails and roads, you'll probably
decide, as most people have, that toe clips aren't appropriate for this kind of riding. So they don't often come on this
kind of bike. All-terrain bikes are sometimes fitted with
longer cranks than conventional bikes (say, 175- or 180-mm
cranks instead of the usual 170s). A different kind of riding
style is evolving for these bikes: slightly higher gears and a
slower cadence combine with the longer cranks to give
you adequate speed and power in the dirt. Of course, the
bike is somewhat slower on pavement than a skinny-tire
dropped-handlebar bike, and this style of pedaling is one
of the reasons why.

On a touring or racing bike, however, you'll probably
want to try toe clips after you've had a few weeks to get
used to the bike. Toe clips come in small, medium and
large sizes, and the sizes are not consistent from one
manufacturer to another. Get toe clips which position your

foot properly, with the ball of your foot over the pedal spindle. If the toe clip is too big, it will allow your foot to slide too far forward on the pedal. If it's the right size, it will snugly hold your foot in the proper position.

Many authors recommend that you buy toe clips which give a quarter to a half inch of space between the front of the shoe and the toe clip. But most riders I know prefer to use the smallest toe clip they can fit into; otherwise they find that their feet move around in that extra space.

Dr. Clifford Graves, medical doctor and veteran cyclist, has told the story of a young French racer who showed great promise but was plagued with a pain in his knees. The cyclist tried hot applications after the race. When that didn't work he went to an orthopedist who performed air injections in the knee joint. The orthopedist suggested doing exercises for the muscles in front of the thigh.

The cyclist followed the doctor's advice but the pain persisted, so he went to a neurologist who gave him tranquilizers and told him to relax. Then to a nutritionist who recommended fruits and vegetables. Then to a psychiatrist who recommended he stop racing.

The racer sold his bike but requested one last ride before he turned it over. On that ride he met a former Tour de France winner and invited him to inspect the bike. The champion looked at the bike and said, "That is a beautiful machine. But your toe clips are too short. Clips like that will cause knee problems."

Saddle Tilt and Fore-Aft Placement.   We must return to the saddle for a couple of simple adjustments. The first is tilt. A saddle with the nose too high will be uncomfortable in some mighty personal areas. A saddle with the nose sloping downward will force the rider to always lean into the handlebars to keep from sliding forward off the saddle.

Accordingly, there is very little variation in proper

saddle position from one cyclist to the next. Most riders like the saddle perfectly parallel to the ground—and that's a good adjustment to try when you're starting out. A few riders like the saddle's nose to point *slightly* up. This helps the rider keep weight off his hands.

If you feel that you have to have your saddle pointing downward, that's a sign that your saddle might be too high. Try lowering the saddle until you are comfortable with its level.

Many people misunderstand saddle fore-aft placement. People often move the saddle far forward (sometimes by turning the seat post clamp around backwards) to put the saddle closer to the handlebars. But when possible, you should adjust the saddle to be in the correct position over the pedals, and then adjust the handlebar stem length to take care of any problems with reach.

All saddle fore-aft placement rules of thumb are designed with position over the pedals in mind. The most accurate rule of thumb is a little difficult to use; you need a friend and a plumb line. Get on the bike in riding position and lean against a wall or doorway so you won't fall over. Put one pedal in the three o'clock (facing forward) position. Have your friend drop the plumb line from the bump on top of your tibia (shinbone). (This bump is just below the kneecap.) The plumb line should fall to the ball of your foot, which is in position directly over the pedal spindle.

If you're of average proportions, you'll be close to this ideal simply by having your saddle in the middle of the seat post clamp. Short people, tall people, and people with long or short thighs may have to make some adjustments to get their saddles where they belong.

Handlebar Position.   Handlebar height is purely a matter of personal preference. Handlebar reach (distance away from you) is not.

Use a handlebar height that you like. Racers like their handlebars very low, so they can bend way over and ride in a compact, aerodynamically efficient position. This position hardly feels comfortable the first time you try it, however, and many people can never get used to it.

If you like your handlebars somewhat higher than the racers have theirs, by all means put them there. You'll put less exotic stress on your back, and you'll find it easier to look around you and signal to other traffic with your bars a bit higher.

Handlebars level with the saddle are considered neutral height; racers have their bars a couple of inches below the saddle; touring cyclists will have their bars at neutral height or an inch or so above.

Your range of options is limited by the sizes of handlebar stems offered for sale. The relevant dimension to handlebar height is *stem column height,* and it doesn't vary much from one manufacturer to the next. The reason is simple: Taller stems break more easily, and manufacturers hate to build anything that might break.

Since you can place your hands anywhere you want on the bars, how you use the bars is a good indication of whether they're an appropriate height for you. If you stay on the tops, try raising the bars. If you keep your elbows straight when you're on the drops, raise the bars a bit. (By the way, always bend your elbows. You can't control the bike smoothly when your elbows are locked straight. It's as bad a habit as locking your legs straight when you're skiing. Bent elbows are an essential part of being able to insulate your pedaling motion from your steering motion.)

Handlebar *reach* must be within a range that allows you to feel relaxed on the bike, so that you can control the bike. Many thousands of people have bikes on which the handlebars are so far away that they never feel in control of the bike, let alone comfortable or relaxed.

Get your friend and your plumb line to see how you

measure up to the reach rule of thumb. Get on the bike with your hands on the drops, arms properly bent as they're supposed to be, feet in position on the pedals, and look ahead, as if you were looking straight down the road. A plumb line dropped from the tip of your nose should land a half inch behind the handlebars.

You may be able to tolerate one or one and a half inches of variation from this rule of thumb; many people can. But many people, particularly short women on frames with long top tubes, are more likely three to five inches away from the rule of thumb. Unhappily, these people often have no choice but to buy a new bike.

If your reach is off, you can change it only by buying a new handlebar stem. Handlebar stems come in extensions from six to fourteen centimeters. Measure your old one (from the center of the column to the center of the handlebars) and add or subtract the centimeters necessary to give the reach you want.

Don't think you have to buy a new stem just because your rule of thumb measurement is a little off. Think about how it would feel, and make the investment only if you expect it would improve your comfort on the bike.

Handlebars also tilt. They should be arranged so the bottom portion is parallel to the ground, or sloping slightly from parallel. Brake levers should be placed where you can feel comfortable grabbing them from above—riding with your hands on the brake hoods is a valuable position, useful for many situations.

Crank Length.   If you're extremely short or extremely tall, you may find the standard 170-mm cranks don't suit you (the crank is the "arm" that supports the pedal). On the other hand, many people find the standard length works okay, and you may as well try to get along with it before undertaking an expensive crankset replacement.

Ed Burke, trainer for the Olympic cycling team, suggests that 170-mm cranks are a good all-around size for most cyclists, though road racers tend to use the 172.5-mm size. Track cyclists tend to use 165s.

Surprisingly, the rules of biomechanics work so that the body is usually more tolerant of changes in crank length than of changes in saddle height, reach, or other factors. I know cyclists ranging from under five feet to over six feet, all of whom are happy with standard length cranks.

But some people cannot ride comfortably unless their cranks are scaled to their bodies. For short people, 165-mm cranks are easy to find. If you hunt and hunt, you may find 150s and 160s. Tall people will find 172.5-, 175-, 177.5- and 180-mm cranks without undue searching. But the 185s craved by so many basketball types are hard to find.

Replacing your cranks is quite expensive, so you'll want to try being happy with the ones that come on the bike.

Frame Size.   Don't skip over this section just because you already own your bike. It's valuable information, because it puts the bike/rider relationship in perspective.

Most Americans are sold bikes by salespersons who ask you to stand over the top tube. If there's an inch of clearance between the top tube and your crotch, you're told that the frame is the right size for you. Usually, this way of sizing customers will result in the customer buying a frame on the large side. There are some significant disadvantages to that.

If you see bike racers, whether in person or in pictures, you'll note that they have very small frames. The seat post is jacked up high. The rider has chosen the smallest frame on which he can get sufficient leg extension.

This allows the racer a lower handlebar position, for better aerodynamics. And the smaller frame is invariably more rigid, which aids in sprinting and hill climbing.

These advantages are the ones cited most often, and they aren't important to a lot of riders. But another advantage is that the smaller frame is easier to handle. You feel more like you're master of the bike on a smaller frame; you can corner better and make more extreme maneuvers.

Should you be using the smallest frame you can fit on, as the racers do? Not necessarily. The racer gives up the option of having the handlebars higher for a more relaxed, easygoing riding position. Since you can't raise the handlebars out of the frame very far, you need a larger frame if you want the handlebars very high. You may want your frame one or two inches larger than the racing-dictated size.

Can your frame be too small? Yes—and you'll know it because you can't get the seat high enough, and/or your hands feel too close in. You can buy extra-long seat posts and 14-cm handlebar stems to "solve" the problem—but with a fix like that, the bike may feel too maneuverable underneath you, like a skateboard.

What if your frame is too large? This can and does happen, as many cyclists like the feel of a big frame, though it likely hampers handling and efficiency. Before you make a decision, get some advice from an experienced cyclist or a bike shop. You can lower the seat, put on shorter cranks and a shorter stem, but you can't change the basic frame. So if it feels too large and appears too large based on the advice I'm giving here, clean it up and get rid of it. Since there is a good market for second-hand bikes, you can probably get a bike shop to take it as a trade-in. Don't compromise your fitness program—and your safety—by riding a frame that doesn't fit you.

Overall Feel. Amateur cyclists at the U.S. Olympic Training Center sometimes simulate real road racing by bumping up against each other. Dangerous? Not really. These racers are not playing a two-wheel game of bumper cars; they are actually learning how to relax on a bike when they are in the middle of a pack moving at 25 to 30 miles per hour. You can imagine the consequences of a lead rider going down or applying his brakes too vigorously going into a turn. Amateur and professional racers must learn to relax on a bike so that when they are in a crowd, they won't become tense.

I'm not suggesting you go out and bump into the first cyclist in sight, but do observe riders in a group. If they are beginners, chances are they will oversteer their bikes and wobble, because they are clinging to their handlebars. If these riders (or their pedals or wheels) touch, more than likely they will go down. If you watch a bike race, especially a criterium—a short race usually held within a city or town—you'll hear the sound of pedal hitting pedal or wheels, though spills are uncommon. Why is this so?

When you are relaxed on a bike, you will literally "go with the flow"; you can be bumped and you will maintain your composure and your balance.

When your bike fits you properly, a number of factors will coincide to make you especially at home on it. When you lean into corners and put weight on one side of the handlebars, a properly sized bike will lean into the corner with you and steer just as much as you want it to. A bike that doesn't fit will oversteer or understeer. Your position over the pedals should feel natural, and it will invite you to work hard—yet it will be just the position you want to be in when you relax and slack off. You'll have several useful hand positions on the bars, and none of them will feel too stretched out or too cramped. By alternating among these positions, you can feel comfortable for hours at a time. Backaches and knee pain will be minimized by your correct position. You'll be able to support much of your weight on your feet and hands, without even realizing that you're doing so, and your fanny will reward you for it by not getting sore.

With proper position on a bike you will be able to accomplish much more, stay in the saddle longer and reap the fitness benefits. Everything follows. Cornering. Climbing and descending hills will be easier and safer. You will find yourself employing techniques that prevent your energy from being drained. You will lay your hands on the handlebars, instead of gripping them tightly. You will keep upper body and torso movement to a minimum, letting your legs do the work. You will learn to anticipate bumps in the road, lifting your buttocks slightly from the saddle. You will move your hands around on the handlebars, as comfort dictates.

You will become master of your bike and your fitness.

4

The Feel of the Pedals

Most recreational cyclists believe that if pedaling doesn't hurt their legs, they are not getting any benefits—a holdover from the "no pain, no gain" school of exercise. The truth of the matter is that easy cycling at a high rpm can return very substantial fitness benefits and actually be less fatiguing, while putting less stress on the muscles.

Pedaling is not like weight lifting; ideally, you should not be pushing down on the pedal, as if against dead weight, but spinning in a circular motion, pulling up on one pedal as you push down on the other (yet another enforcement for toe clips).

Scientific studies and the experience of expert cyclists point to this conclusion: You'll ride faster, farther and develop better cardiovascular endurance, by using a lower gear, spinning the pedals quickly, and having a lighter pressure on each pedal. That is a rule of thumb you should internalize and live with.

Beginning cyclists often find this style of riding takes some getting used to. They're used to pushing hard on each pedal stroke. The idea that a light, almost effortless pedal stroke could be good exercise seems suspicious. And, most of all, beginners have trouble spinning the pedals smoothly. It takes little coordination to spin pedals at 40 rpm or so, as many riders do. But you want to train your legs to spin comfortably at more than twice that speed, and that takes some practice.

How do you know how fast you're spinning? Most people count. On a quiet stretch of road, see how many pedal revolutions you turn over in 15 seconds. Multiply that by four, and you have your cadence—your pedaling rate in rpm. If you count your cadence often enough, you'll begin to learn what various cadences feel like, so you'll be able to know by feel about how fast you're going.

There is a high-tech alternative to this way of measuring your cadence. Some of the electronic bicycle speedometers now offered for sale have cadence functions. If you invest in one of those, you'll be able to find your exact cadence at the push of a button. However, all these electronic speedometers with cadence functions are expensive—more than $50, and usually a lot more—so you may decide that counting cadence on a quiet road is a good alternative. At any event I'll discuss the cadence meter in greater detail in Chapter Five.

As I stated earlier, you want to develop your legs so they can spin comfortably at a brisk cadence of around 90 rpm. The cadence just right for you may not be the same as for your friends. Larger, more muscular people may opt for slightly slower cadences (say, 85 rpm—or even 80 for a very big rider) and smaller, thinner people may find spinning at 95 or even 100 rpm most comfortable. Whatever your natural cadence is, there are two elements you must keep in mind to work up to it:

1. You should pedal at progressively quicker cadences as your body develops the ability to handle them smoothly, and

2. You need to do some practicing at cadences faster than your natural cadence so that your legs are really at home when you pedal at your natural cadence.

If you're a 40-rpm slogger, plan on spending two or three weeks to change your habits to a high-cadence rider. During these weeks, do all your riding in low gears that seem ridiculously easy. If this seems silly or Mickey Mouse to you, relax. You're in good company. The top European professional racers, who regularly ride more than 150 miles per day at speeds above 25 miles per hour, start their training with a thousand miles of low-gear spinning at easy effort. It is only then the professional starts pushing big gears.

Put your bike in a gear that feels easy (the next chapter covers gearing in more detail). Ride at a cadence that feels brisk. You should feel as though you're only pressing very lightly on the pedals. If you have to push hard on the pedals, downshift. Keep your legs spinning briskly.

Be conscious of your riding style—and partners. It is very easy to get caught up in someone else's pace or gearing. Smother the inclination to race or ride on someone's wheel early in your training. That will come in time. For the time being, get to know your bike and yourself.

If you're not used to spinning, you may find this kind of workout fatiguing in an unaccustomed way: Your legs don't get tired from the effort of pushing the pedals, but they get tired from the effort of moving their own weight around. That's to be expected. Your legs are learning the coordination of spinning—and this is just like learning how to throw a fast ball, or how to dance a fancy step. It takes practice for the body to learn how to do it right. At first, it will take more mental effort on your part; but as you go on, you'll find that your legs learn to spin by themselves. You'll get smoother too. Your upper body will remain still as your legs churn like eggbeaters at quick cadences. You'll enjoy the way your newfound skill allows you to accelerate away from stoplights, or scoot up hills, while you remain rock steady, composed and smooth in the saddle.

At first, you'll probably find that a cadence of 60 or 70 is as fast as you can handle. If you don't have the clips on your bike, you'll reach your ceiling very quickly: 75 or so is as fast as you'll be able to spin. If you do have toe clips, a little mental effort will train your body to spin faster and faster, until you find a 90-rpm cruising cadence quite natural.

How much faster than 90 rpm should you force yourself to experiment with in training? That depends on your goals as a cyclist. If you want to race, you'll need to learn to sprint, and sprint well—and that calls for practicing cadences up to 150, so you can sprint at 130 or 140 while staying smooth enough to control the bike. (These figures may sound awesome, but they're not an upper extreme. Many racers take this even further, and train their legs to 180+ rpm.) If sprinting doesn't interest you, you'll probably find that a cadence of 110 or so is as fast as you ever need to train at.

Moreover, if your main goal is to enjoy getting fit through cycling, you won't want to make your workouts dreary by worrying too much about your maximum sprint rpm. If you don't find that aspect of cycling pleasurable for its own sake, don't dwell on it. Above all, the idea is to have fun doing something that's good for you.

As you increase your cadence, you should be particularly attentive to the gears you are using. Lower your optimum gears if it helps you spin. As I will discuss more fully later, you might want to strengthen your leg muscles with leg presses and leg curls. You might want to do this anyway for overall strength.

To a cetain extent spinning at an even cadence is partly a fiction—a necessary fiction—because, though you might be turning the left and right cranks an equal number of times, you are probably not delivering the same amount of power to the pedals. The reason for this phenomenon is that, whether we know it or not, one leg is stronger than the other. I was surprised that, when I was measured by a computer hooked up to a bicycle at the Pennsylvania State Biomechanical Laboratory, my left leg was found to be significantly weaker than the right. I later duplicated the results at the Shimano Biomechanical Testing Center in Japan. I shouldn't have been surprised, as most cyclists, both competitive and recreational, enjoy this deficiency.

Rebecca Twigg, a likely gold medalist for the U.S. in the road race in the 1984 Olympics, learned in tests at Penn State that her left leg was 20 percent stronger than her right, so she started a weight-training program to compensate. Similar tests on 50 recreational cyclists showed that most of them pedaled predominantly with one leg. Peter Cavanagh, Ph.D., director of the Biomechanics Lab, suggested recreational cyclists exaggerate the action of each leg so they get a sense of what asymmetrical pedaling feels like. He also suggested weight training.

Keep in mind that pedaling per se is not a very efficient action. Cavanaugh notes that,

> In our studies, we found that only 50 percent of the [recreational cyclist's] applied force is used efficiently in the production of external work (such as turning the pedal). That's simply because the circular mechanics is a very inefficient one. It's just an inefficient way of coupling the person to the back wheel because in certain times in the cycle you cannot apply large forces at right angles to the crank, which is what you need to do.

In Chapter Five I'll talk about ways to improve your pedaling and cadence. For now just be conscious of your spin and the force you apply to the pedals. Think and pedal circles. Though the action won't deliver much power to the rear wheel, pull up on your toe clips as you go through the recovery phase (after you reach the bottom of the downstroke). Try not to think of the pedaling action as a push-pull process, as that will encourage you to apply maximum force on the downstroke and ease up on the upstroke. Be aware of the roundness of your pedaling until it becomes second nature. That kind of cycling will not only take you farther, it will also enable you to be comfortable and efficient while getting fit.

5

Maintaining Cadence

I once overheard a conversation between twelve-year-olds about gearing. One argued that since he had 18 speeds he could go faster than the other who had a measly 12 speeds. I didn't wait around for the outcome because I have heard so many similar exchanges. I purchased for my son, aged eleven, a 10-speed which had exactly that number of gearing options. My son felt at a distinct disadvantage to his mother, who had an 18-speed. More means faster and so it goes.

The linking of multiple gears and raw speed, held in the consumer's mind like a matched pair, has been generously fostered by the bicycle industry which in a few short years has offered bikes with 10, 12, 15, 18 and 21 "gears," promising speed and a phenomenal number of choices.

If you have a bicycle with ten distinct and usable gears, you could probably handle most terrains. Consider Tour de France riders who rarely use more than a six-cog cluster even when climbing the Alps. And these are professionals for whom the difference of a couple of teeth on the rear cog can affect the outcome of a race.

Whether you need 18 gears or more or less, is up to you. But you certainly need a range of gearing on your bike because even very modest hills slow you down considerably. For example, a two-percent grade, which climbs two feet in a hundred, will slow you down about 6 mph if you maintain your effort. If you're breezing along at 18 mph, that's a 30 percent decrease in speed, significant in any vehicle. The transmission in your car would sneer at a two-percent grade, but not so your bike; you should indeed shift gears for that slight increase in elevation.

By now you should be relaxed on a bike and used to the feel of the pedals. Your emphasis has been on high rpm cycling, and your body is probably used to that kind of rhythm. You'll notice some disadvantages if you vary your cadence by more than ten percent. If you pedal too slowly, your legs will quickly feel heavy. If you pedal too fast, you will expend most of your energy just fanning the pedals. The way to keep your cadence smooth and steady is by choosing the right gearing to match the terrain.

Gearing involves cogs and chainwheels and mechanical advantage expressed in ratios and inches. In this chapter I will discuss how to make the most of your gearing to maintain optimum cadence. Part I is reasonably simple and straightforward and I encourage you to read it right away. Part II is a little more complicated, as it's an introduction to the complicated world of analyzing and improving your bike's gearing.

Depending on how you feel about numbers and technical matters, you might want to skip Part II now and come back to it after reading Chapter Eleven, Your Championship Form. If you find that the gearing on your bike meets your needs, ignore Part II. But as you become a more experienced rider, sensitive to the nuances of your bike, you may want a more discriminating gear selection. Like professional and amateur racers, you might be able to differentiate between two cogs that are a tooth apart.

I. INTRODUCTION TO GEARING

Your bike has so many speeds (10, 12, 18) so that you can select the right ratio for the exact terrain, headwind and legpower of the moment, and have a broad enough range of ratios to handle everything from steep uphills to steep downhills.

There's one wrinkle in this logic: The selection of ratios on most bikes is quite poor, and it's difficult to learn to use it. Sometimes it's so bad that you'll want to replace it. Consequently, you will want to learn about gear ratios on bikes in general, and how to apply them to understand the gearing on your bike, and then decide whether the gearing suits your needs.

First, though, we'll go through the basics without getting too analytical about it. Most bikes have two front sprockets, called chainwheels, and five or six rear sprockets, called cogs. On most bikes, the larger chainwheel is about an inch larger in radius than the smaller chainwheel. The way most cyclists use the gearing is to use the small chainwheel for hill climbing and for easy day riding; the large chainwheel is for flats and downhills on hard-riding days. The cyclist uses the rear derailleur for fine tuning; small cogs for downhills, larger cogs for uphills.

There are many possible variations to this way of using the gears, and cyclists who like mathematics often spend hours thinking about them. Entire societies have sprung up around this arcane science. However, for now, it's not important that you worry about that. The most important thing for you to do is to practice using the derailleurs quickly, crisply, and without hesitation. Remember, your "engine" works poorly if you're pedaling too slow or too fast. So you want to learn to anticipate when you'll need to shift, so you shift at (or even a second before) the moment you need to, rather than as an afterthought.

Think of it this way: An unskilled cyclist knows when to shift only by noticing that his legs are spinning much too fast or too slow. A skilled cyclist not only stays alert for much smaller variations in cadence, he also anticipates shifting needs by looking at the terrain ahead. That cyclist will always be spinning at the correct cadence, which requires practice and anticipation.

You have to be skilled at manipulating your derailleurs. It's not difficult to learn this skill, but if you don't, you'll never think in terms of shifting ahead. If it's difficult for you to shift, you'll tend to avoid shifting, and you'll avoid thinking about shifting.

So if you don't like to think about shifting, spend 20 minutes now and then practicing it. Go to an empty parking lot or quiet dead-end street, where you're free from distractions. Teach yourself to shift up one cog, then down one cog, then up one cog, etc. Keep doing that so that it feels more natural. Observe what happens when you have to shift lower. When you're actually riding the bike, you want to shift one cog at a time, most of the time. You may occasionally want to shift two cogs at a time. So you don't want to be the cyclist who knows only how to shift all five or six at once, or maybe an unknown number (two to four, but you're never sure). You want to have better control over your derailleurs than that. With some practice, it will feel completely natural, and then you won't have to think about it anymore. It will be like driving a stick shift.

If you read this far and practice what we preach, you'll be doing pretty well—much better than 99 percent of the people who sometimes ride bikes. If you read further, you'll start to climb the ranks within the final one percent— the people who really get their money's worth out of all ten speeds, people who really use their bikes as a fitness tool.

Gearing is always discussed in gear inches. (The French use a metric-system-based alternative measure, called *development,* but never mind that.) Gear inches date back to when manufacturers of the so-called safety bicycle were trying to advertise their wares in competition with the high-wheeler or ordinary bike. High-wheelers had always been sold by the wheel diameter. A child would ride a high-wheeler with about a 36-inch diameter. An adult would ride one about 45 inches in diameter, perhaps a bit bigger if the rider had long legs. The bigger a wheel you could straddle on one of those things, the farther you would go with each turn of the pedals (since one turn of the pedals equaled one turn of the wheel) and the faster you could ride.

The safety bicycle, with its much smaller wheels and chain drive, had to be sold to cyclists who were used to buying bikes by wheel diameter. So manufacturers multiplied the wheel diameter of their new bikes by the gear ratio that the chain drive had, which was one of the first advertising initiatives in the bike industry. This new figure, called gear inches, told the customer what size wheel on an ordinary bike the safety bike could correspond to.

In other words,

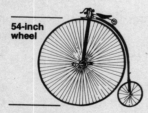

One revolution of the pedals

takes you as far as

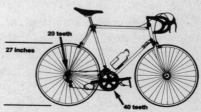

One revolution of the pedals

The short formula for gear inches looks like this:

$$\text{Gear Inches} = \text{Rear Wheel Diameter} \times \frac{\text{number of front chainwheel teeth}}{\text{number of rear cog teeth}}$$

So, if you have a 27-inch rear wheel, a 40-tooth chainwheel and a 20-tooth rear cog, your gear inches look like this:

$$\text{Gear Inches} = 27 \times \frac{40}{20}$$

$$= 27 \times 2$$

$$= 54$$

Of course, if your bike has five rear cogs and two chainwheels, you have ten possible combinations. You count how many teeth are on each cog and chainwheel, and write down the gear inches on a chart like this:

	40	52 Chainwheel teeth
14	77	100
17	63	83
20	54	70
24	45	59
28	38	50

Rear cog teeth (left of table, rows 20 and 24)

Gear inches

Make a small chart like this one, and tape it to your handlebars. It will help you remember what the various gears on your bike feel like, and with its help you'll always know what gear you're in, and what a shift would feel like. In time, you'll have a pretty good feel for what gear you're in, without actually looking down through your legs at the cogs.

As you can see, on the bike from which my example chart was taken, the gear inches range from 38 on the easiest gear to 100 on the hardest gear. Here's what the range of gear inches is best used for:

20 inches	Steep uphills with bike bags
30 inches	Steep uphills
40 inches	Somewhat steep uphills
50 inches	Moderate uphills
60 inches	Easy riding on level ground or slight uphills
70 inches	Brisk riding on level ground
80 inches	Hard riding on level ground, or slight downhills
90 inches	Sprinting on level ground, or moderate downhills
100 inches	Somewhat steep downhills
110 inches	Unsafe speeds on steep downhills

These ranges represent a rule of thumb that you can apply to your own riding style. Consider them a place to start.

The sample chart shows the way many 10-speed bikes are geared as they come from the factory. (I've been lecturing the bike industry for years on this subject.) Note that the low gear is 38 inches, which is probably not low enough for steep hills, according to the chart. That's why you see so many people pushing 10-speed bikes up hills— they can't pedal comfortably with the gearing provided. When these people try a good touring bike with a 25-inch gear, they're delighted. The whole world seems flat again. So many cyclists would be well served if their bikes had lower gears.

At the other extreme, a 100-inch gear is quite high. If you were strong enough to pedal it at the cadence of 90 rpm recommended some pages ago (and almost no cyclist is that strong) you would be cruising at 27 mph! Since speeds greater than that are frequently unsafe, there's little need to equip your bike to attain them.

II. OTHER GEARING OPTIONS

Already, you may be wondering whether you would profit from a higher high gear or a lower low gear on your own bike. But surprisingly you're more likely to find that you'd profit from a change in the middle gears. Here's why: On many bikes, the middle gears are so poorly positioned that you can't maintain your cadence as evenly as you'd like to.

Here's a specific example, drawn from my example gearing: Suppose you're on flat road with a tailwind, and you're pedaling at 90 rpm in the 83-inch gear. (You'll be going 22 mph.) Ninety is as fast as you want to spin, but you could push a slightly higher gear with help from that tailwind. Your next higher gear is 100 inches. Shift into it, and your cadence immediately drops to 76. That's much too slow, and it feels bad to your feet. So you push harder, and accelerate the bike one-and-a-half mph to 23½ mph. (This is a big increase in speed! Wind resistance makes each mile per hour much more work to attain than the one before it.) Your cadence is still only 79 rpm.

There you have it: Shift down to the 83-inch gear, and it's too low. The 100-inch gear is too high. A gear in the middle would be perfect. (And it would be more all-around useful than your 100-inch gear.) So, you could choose to sacrifice your 100-inch gear by having a bike shop replace your 14-tooth small cog with a 15-tooth cog. Then you'd have a 94-inch gear in place of the 100-inch gear.

This change solves one problem, but it creates another. It's worth learning what this problem is, so that you'll be on the lookout for similar problems that may occur if you change the gearing on your own bike. Remembering all this talk about gearing has a physiological dimension: The right gearing will help you pedal more efficiently, which is the cornerstone of fitness through cycling.

The problem is this: When you change the 14-tooth cog, you affect not only the 100-inch high gear, but also the 77-inch "eighth" gear. Cyclists seldom use the designations "seventh," "eighth," etc., because the shift pattern makes it hard to figure out exactly how the gears are ranked.

On this particular bike, the 77-inch gear was perfectly positioned between the 70-inch gear and the 83-inch gear. Shifting among these three gears would give you the small changes you want to maintain exactly the cadence you want. (The 77-inch gear's position on the gear chart grid isn't very handy; you have to make two shifts to get at it from the 83-inch gear, and three to get at it from the 70-inch gear. Across once and up once; across once and up twice! But the gear does exist for cyclists who are willing to reach for it.)

If you change the 14-tooth cog to a 15-tooth, the 77-inch gear becomes a 72-inch gear—a near-exact duplicate of the 70-inch gear. Now you have a too large gap between your 70-inch gear and your 83-inch gear. There's no free lunch.

There are some specific solutions to this problem, and I'll get to them in a minute. But first, you want to look at some of the general principles that this problem illustrates.

Many riders won't find this a problem at all. Many riders aren't fussy enough about their cadence to need to make such fine shifts. You may be one of them. If so, please proceed to the next chapter. Or you may find that you don't need to make fine shifts now, but after a season of serious training, you'll want to. If so, hang in there.

I could fill this book with gear charts and suggested possible combinations of chainwheel teeth and rear cog teeth. You would probably find that boring. So instead, here are the considerations you'll want to keep in mind:

On the example given (page 52), the bike was designed so that all the large chainwheel gears are coordinated with the small chainwheel gears. Each adjacent gear is "across and up" or "across and down." If you rank them in order, they look like this:

	40	52 Chainwheel teeth
14	8	10
17	6	9
20	4	7
24	2	5
28	1	3

Rear cog teeth (label for the first column: 14, 17, 20, 24, 28)

To shift from third to fourth, you have to move the chain from the large chainwheel to the small one, and the chain from the outermost cog to the third one in. Then, if you want to go into fifth gear, you'll have to put the chain back on the large chainwheel and drop down a cog. And so on. You can put those shifts on the gear chart on your handlebars.

This is every bit as complicated as it looks! Few cyclists ever bother to make the double- and triple-shifts necessary to work their way through this maze. Instead, they make do with the gears available through single shifts.

This particular arrangement is called *alpine* gearing. The name implies gearing for hilly country, but in that sense it's a misnomer. It doesn't give you a very low hill-climbing gear. Any alpine gearing setup will have a large gap between the top gear and the second-to-the-top gear. (Theoretically, there's another large gap between the bottom gear and the second-to-the-bottom gear, but in practice, that gap doesn't matter.) If you bought your bike in the past couple years, it may have a 12-speed version of alpine gearing, perhaps with 42/52 chainwheels and a 14-16-19-22-26-30 freewheel. The advantage of a 12-speed alpine is that the smaller jumps on the freewheel make it more pleasant to pedal when you don't bother with the exotic shift pattern.

Forget alpine. Many cyclists prefer to arrange their gearing so that there is no coordination between large chainwheel gears and small chainwheel gears. They use the large chainwheel for flats and downhills, and the small chainwheel for uphills and relaxed pedaling. Fine-tuning shifts are made on the rear derailleur. This setup is called *crossover*.

Easy shifting makes this kind of setup convenient. There's only one disadvantage: You don't get 10 (or 12) distinct gears. You're likely to get lots of duplications. But if the bike works well, the duplications aren't really a problem. The fact is that you can get a good workout with 6 to 7 available gears.

This kind of setup, by the way, is the best solution for most people who want to solve the alpine problem I presented earlier. For example, you could replace your freewheel with a 14-15-17-19-22-26 freewheel. The gaps between adjacent cogs on this freewheel are small enough to satisfy a constant cadence fan. If you put this on your alpine-geared bike, you make the shifting easier, and you wind up with a slight change in your lowest gear.

There are many other solutions that would enable you to have 10 or 12 useful gears, but I don't need to go into them at this time. The important thing for you to remember is that the secret to effective cycling is for you to maintain a level of cadence and rpm, no matter the terrain. How you accomplish this is through proper gearing.

You've seen that most factory equipped bikes usually have a gear that is too high, and one that is not low enough. Let's face it, you can certainly get by with that kind of gearing and get a good workout. What you will also get—frequently—are large jumps between gears, especially in the middle ranges. As you cycle you will find that your pedaling will fall off or speed up significantly because of these jumps. But you can live with that system. And get fit in the process.

As suggested, you could ask your bike shop to replace your 14-tooth cog with a 15-tooth. That would get rid of your 100 gear, but you'd also lose a middle gear (a 77-inch).

You'll have to ask yourself whether the other solutions are worth your time. The double-shift gearing arrangement offers smaller jumps between gears but demands a lot of shifting. If you don't want to bother with this, consider a 12-speed gearing that permits single shifts. Or consider crossover gearing. Though this system will give you fewer gears, you'll find it easier to use. I've been using this system on one of my bikes for years and have never felt at a severe disadvantage when cycling with others who had more gears at their disposal. They shifted more than I did and probably pedaled more efficiently.

I recommend you spend a few minutes counting the number of teeth on your chainwheel and cogs and work up your gear chart to paste on your handlebars, especially if you are a beginning cyclist. Sure, you'll get your hands dirty, but once and for all it will take the mystery out of those strange moving parts.

Through inspection, you can pretty well tell if you have gears that overlap—meaning they are too close in gear-inch numbers to provide added benefit. If that is the case, you might choose to live with it or choose one of the alternatives offered here. The simplest way to do that is to visit your local bike shop, explain your situation and needs. Spending a few dollars to get a more satisfactory gearing arrangement might, in the long run, be well worth the money.

At this point in your development, don't think of the gearing in mechanical terms. Think of it as the way for you to get maximum benefit from your bike and your body. Your bike's a tool for fitness. Start out with the right arrangement of moving parts and your body will feel the difference.

6

A Good Workout

America has been nourished on the notion that for a routine to be considered exercise, it must have matriculated in the push-and-pull school of rigor and gruel. To be exercise, something has to hurt. To be beneficial one must engage an immovable force, much like Sisyphus, who pushed rocks for a living.

At various gatherings and on various platforms, often dwarfed by real athletes from the hard-hitting sports, I've spoken about cycling as "soft" exercise. Over the manly groans of the audience I've explained that by "soft," I surely don't mean that cycling doesn't make you work; on the contrary, performed properly, cycling is one of the most demanding aerobic activities. By "soft" I mean a rhythmic, cardiovascular exercise that is kind to your weight-bearing joints, especially the knees.

To get the most out of your bicycle and the most out of yourself, you'll likely have to rethink your perception of exercise. On a bike you are not simply pushing against resistance, as in weight training, or moving yourself through space in a quick time; you are moving a biomechanical "unit" across varying terrain at a pace that will safely and surely condition your legs and lungs. And done properly, there will be no strain and no pain.

Early-Season Low-Gear Training. Those who have followed the Tour de France know that the race is probably the most arduous sporting event in the world, lasting for more than 20 days and 2,000 miles. (I confess I am beginning to wonder whether the Race Across America, a nonstop contest from coast to coast in under 10 days, isn't a close rival.)

How do the great professional riders in Europe begin their training for a tough, competitive season? Softly, with more than a thousand miles of low-gear training. Often in training these racers will use a single-speed, fixed-gear bike which eliminates coasting. When the wheels move, so do the pedals (I discuss this option in detail in Chapter Eighteen).

Fixed-gear training, while not essential for the recreational cyclist, does have some benefits. Since the pedals turn with the wheels, there's no freewheeling, you don't cheat. Furthermore, you are forced to develop a smooth, even spin, rather than just pushing down on the pedals. You work every inch of the way.

You won't know until you are further along on cycling whether a fixed gear would benefit you. Chances are that, if you catch the bug and want to join the amateur ranks for your age group, you will make the investment. But for now, you can earn all the benefits of fixed-gear training by staying in low gears.

The whole idea behind low-gear training is that you can't go fast, an urge that most of us find hard to resist, particularly on that sunny Sunday in March when spring seems close at hand. The point is: You don't *want* to go fast. At a cadence of 90 in a 60-inch gear you'll only be going 16 mph. Now is the time to concentrate on turning the pedals, pedaling in circles, rather than squares.

When that breath of spring raises your adrenaline, you don't just shift and push harder; you spin faster. Each time you try for a quicker cadence than before, teaching your legs a new sense of coordination.

High-rpm, low-gear training is meant to develop your aerobic endurance. You are gradually stressing your muscles, tendons, and ligaments. Later in the season you will get the muscle strength from other specific workouts.

You can start these early-season rides by going somewhat short distances, say, six to ten miles. There's no need to overwhelm your winter legs with too many miles too soon. (If you were one of those European professionals, daily mileage would start out at 30 to 40 miles.)

You'll quickly discover one aspect of early-season low-gear training; because it's slow and somewhat easy, it can be boring. Take pains to avoid that. Ride with friends, make a picnic out of it, explore new byways. Note that you can take advantage of low-gear riding's slower speed to be sociable and ride with friends who may not be tenacious cyclists. They may make fun of your churning legs, but never mind that. You'll have the last laugh.

You'll probably feel pumped up and vigorous after low-gear rides, instead of feeling soggy and worn out. There's a benefit you don't get with early-season training in most sports! The low-gear training forces your heart and lungs to work hard, pumping your body full of oxygen-rich blood. Your muscles, which haven't been straining against too-high resistance, will still have some life left in them.

This may lead you to suspect that you haven't had much of a workout. Don't believe it. You'll see that it was a good workout by other signs—how mellow you feel late in the day, and how well you sleep that night. Your heart and lungs, your blood vessels, and the digestive system that feeds them have all been taxed heavily. You haven't been pounding your bones or straining your leg muscles, but you've been working hard on the body systems which are the core of high level fitness. With cycling, fitness will sneak up on you.

Before you tell yourself it's time to graduate from early-season low-gear training, roll up a significant number of miles this way. A serious racer would want 1,000 to 1,500 low-gear (and possibly fixed-gear) miles pedaled in four to six weeks before entering the next stage of training. You may settle for less. Less serious racers I've known will get off the fixed-and-low-gear after around 200 miles. (Even 75 miles—five ten-mile rides and one 25-mile ride—will make a huge difference in how the rest of your training unfolds.) It'll make your pedaling smoother, and it will teach you to listen to your leg muscles and sense how hard they're working. It will help you stop bouncing in the saddle, so that your entire upper body remains rock steady while your legs spin. It will give your leg muscles the coordination to put more of their energy into spinning the pedals, and less energy into fighting each other.

Train, Don't Strain.   The next stage in your training is the move to medium-size gears. Allow yourself the luxury of gears up to about 75 inches on level roads, using higher and lower gears as terrain dictates. At this stage, be careful to maintain a brisk cadence; it's quite easy to slide into a slow cadence/high gear habit, and you'll have to make a conscious effort to avoid doing so. Practice keeping an eye on the wristwatch you've strapped to your handlebars as you count pedal revolutions to allow you to keep tabs on your cadence. If you splurge and buy an electronic speedometer with a cadence function, keeping track of cadence will be downright fun. It will also keep you honest.

At this point in your training, you still should avoid worrying about your overall average miles per hour. The average will be a bit on the low side, since your self-imposed gearing ceiling keeps you from going as fast on the flats as you otherwise could. That's okay, because you're still not ready to push monster-high gears. You're still learning how your legs feel as they spin.

If you allow yourself too-high gears at this point, you'll find that you can spin them and ride fast for a fairly short distance—a mile or less—and then you'll feel worn out. You want to avoid this, because it will lead you to ride unevenly, interspersing hard and easy periods. You have to learn how to maintain a steady, well-paced effort first. *Train, don't strain.*

By keeping your legs churning and avoiding coasting, you'll get a lot of exercise value out of this style of riding, even if your time on the bike is limited by worldly obligations. The slightly higher gears will make your leg muscles stronger—particularly since you've prepared for them with your low-gear training. The constant motion of your legs will bring you cardiovascular fitness. The relatively light amount of strain you're putting on your knees and tendons will allow them to adapt gradually to the stresses of cycling, instead of becoming injured from overuse and causing you misery.

If time permits, you should ride distances up to 50 miles (or even more, should you be so ambitious) in the moderate-gear mode. These extra-long workouts have a benefit you'll never get from any combination of shorter workouts: They train your body for endurance by changing the way your muscles burn fuel. Muscles that aren't trained for endurance burn glycogen, the "high octane" fuel in your bloodstream. That's okay, but your body has a limited amount of glycogen. Even a well-trained athlete has only about two hours' worth of glycogen to draw on. When the glycogen is all gone, your muscles have to burn fat—and your body has to get used to that.

If you're trying to shed a few pounds, the benefits of having your muscles burn fat should be obvious. But your body doesn't automatically shift from burning glycogen to burning fat. Unless you train it to burn fat, it will only do so with difficulty.

It's hard to miss the signs that you've switched from

glycogen to fat. You'll be in the midst of a long ride and your verve will disappear. You'll find yourself needing low gears *and* a low cadence, since your body will be limping along with little energy. You'll hurt. You'll also want to ride straight home without stopping, since you'll sense that if you get off the bike, you won't want to climb back on.

As you train more and more for endurance, burning fat won't feel so bad. Your body will adapt to burn fat more efficiently, and it will actually learn to burn some fat at the beginning of the workout, particularly during the low-effort warm-up miles. You'll use fat for steady efforts and glycogen for sprints and climbs. This stretches your glycogen supply considerably.

The benefits of this endurance training are a joy to experience. You can be out on a very long ride—a club century (100-miler) for instance—and, even late in the ride, have the extra energy to pounce up every hill. It feels eerie, and quite pleasant, to have this kind of energy left after you've expended so much already.

A three-hour total workout every week or every other week is the bare minimum you'd need to start realizing these fast-burning benefits. If you can spare the time, do it. If you can't, good cardiovascular fitness isn't such a bad consolation prize.

A month or two of medium-gear training with some long rides thrown in will, in combination with the early-season low-gear training, give you a solid base on which to build exotic fitness. A recreational cyclist will need to train about 200 miles per month as a bare minimum to build a good foundation. If your goals are more ambitious than recreational cycling, the mileage must be too. To comfortably complete multiday loaded tours and club centuries, you'll want a base with more mileage in it—100 miles per week would be good for many riders. A competitive racer would want to double this figure.

After you've built a good base this way, you can actually maintain it with less time spent on the bike. The base will give you the ability to train hard, so that you can go out for short rides and really burn during those relatively short rides.

Interval Training. This brings us to the next stage of training—"really burning"—when you glue your nose to the handlebar stem and spin furiously in large (85-to-90-inch) gears. After you've built your fitness base, you'll be aching for the chance to show off some of your newfound fitness this way.

Now you'll be ready to ride intervals—medium duration bursts of more intense effort. In the early season, intervals would leave you gasping for air and courting stress injury, but now they're a rewarding challenge. After a half hour to an hour of warm-up on easy terrain, you ride at high effort for one to three minutes. (If you don't like looking at a watch, count 15 telephone poles for your interval distance.) Ride easily for a recovery period of a couple minutes, then repeat the interval. If you want to quit after two or three, you rode too hard. You should be able to do a half dozen before taking the shortcut home.

Intervals send your pulse a-pounding, and the intense heartbeat and breathing they force upon you may cause discomfort. (Obviously, if you experience serious pains, particularly in the chest, and they persist, see your doctor.) An interval workout is something to be conquered, and you will sooner or later develop the ability to ride a hard interval workout without undue discomfort.

One thing about riding intervals is that it's hard to know how fast you're going, and whether you're progressing from week to week. Runners and swimmers clock their laps with a stopwatch, and their workout schedules place a great deal of emphasis on the exact time each interval should take. It's not so convenient to do that on a bike.

Even track riders on the velodrome, where each lap is a set distance, don't make much use of lap times. They're riding too fast to hear the manager read the times off the watch.

This may strike you as a drawback. How are you supposed to know if you're improving, if you don't know how fast you're going? Well, one of the purposes of the early-season cycling was to help you get to know the feel of your bike so well that you could sense whether you're going faster or not. But beyond that, there are two possible solutions.

The first, and more traditional, solution is to ride intervals with a group of like-minded cyclists. You'll help challenge each other, and you'll see how you compare with each other from week to week. This is a valuable and important bonus. Group riding will help you ride harder and attain greater fitness for the same level of mental effort.

The second solution is to join the electronic age and buy an electronic speedometer/cadence meter. Then your interval can become more digital; you ride for two minutes at 105 rpm, or at 24 mph, or whatever you please. If you have the money, one of these little toys can make your training much more systematic.

Intervals can be of different styles, for different purposes. You may want to vary the duration of the effort period, working harder on days when you've selected a one-minute effort and not as hard on days when you've selected a three-minute effort. You can put the bike in the biggest gear you can briefly get a good spin out of (say, 90 to 95 inches) and really burn out your legs to develop strength. You can use a medium-high gear (85 inches) and go for a combination of speed and duration. You can use a lower gear (75 to 80 inches) and work on your snap. Racers do this all the time. If you don't race and don't care about being the fastest one away from the stoplight, you may not want to do this kind of interval. But it's available if you do.

Another trick is to vary your interval workout. You can mix one-minute high-effort periods with two-minute semi-high-effort periods. You can alternate big chainwheel intervals and small chainwheel intervals, getting both a strength workout and a snap workout on the same day.

Of course, you can't do any hard workout day after day. When you've had a hard workout, ride gently for a day or two to recover. Even if your legs aren't sore, as they would be after a hard running workout, your body is exhausted and needs the rest.

Hills. One thing that's unavoidable for most riders is climbing hills. Many experienced riders prefer to avoid hills during the early season, since hills interfere with the easy-pedaling strategy. If your bike is equipped with wide-range touring gearing, however, that won't be a problem. Use your 30-inch gear, and your 25-inch gear if the bike has one, and enjoy your gentle early-season conditioning on the most scenic mountains you can climb.

Later in the season, the hills will still be there. How you approach them is a matter of personal preference. Many riders, particularly committed long-distance tourists, like to stay in the saddle, gear down, and spin while the bike inches its way to the summit. Racers and would-be racers are more likely to get out of the saddle and impatiently jump from pedal to pedal, urging the bike onward in a gear much higher than the tourist would use. And some riders switch their approach from week to week, depending on their mood.

You may have your own ideas about how you'd like to ride hills. There are some limitations, however. If you have the slightest hint of knee trouble, a stand-up-and-honk style will be very hard on your knees. If you're touring with panniers, you'll find standing and honking slow, exhausting, even harder on your knees, and much less productive than it is on an unloaded bike. People simply aren't made strong enough to ride that way on loaded bikes. For either of these kinds of riders, a leisurely climbing style is indicated. A racer has no choice. The field climbs hard and fast, with the lightweight riders moving to the front to force the pace and drop the poorer climbers.

Many riders climb slowly because they never learn to pace themselves on long, steady climbs. Again, the early-season training may help you to do that. But pacing is more difficult on a climb. Your momentum disappears if you slack off even for an instant, and the bike needs a more steady power input. It takes practice to get the feel of putting power into the bike that steadily, and it also takes practice to feel around for your aerobic limit so you can ride as fast as you can without "blowing up."

Practice will make you a smoother climber. Picking the right gear, anticipating when to shift, pedaling smoothly and staying just inside your aerobic limit will all get you to the top quicker. And all require on-the-bike practice.

Time Trials. Just as some bike riders never climb very quickly, others never go very fast on the flats. And the differences are usually more a matter of practice and finesse than of raw aerobic ability. Sure, a small, light guy has an advantage in climbing. But there are plenty of big, tall riders who climb better than they go on the flats.

Fast riding on the flats, particularly when you're doing it by yourself, is thought of as *time trialing* by many cyclists. Time trialing, of course, is a racing event in which the cyclist rides alone, unpaced, completing an assigned distance against the clock. The riding style that this event demands is punishing, but it sure is fun to go that fast. With 1,000 or 2,000 training miles behind you for the season, you can tuck your nose to the handlebar stem, select an 85-inch or 90-inch gear, and ride at a near-25-mph clip for a 25-mile time trial.

If you want to ride this fast, you'll quickly discover that an aerodynamic position on the bike is very important. Hands on the drops, back bent over, arms bent . . . when you stick your head up just enough to sneak a quick sip from your water bottle, you'll feel the increased air resistance slowing you down.

Accordingly, you want to learn to ride mile after mile, comfortably, in a good aerodynamic position. This is, at best, an acquired taste. Even in road races, many riders assume a less efficient position, and casual time trialists accept slower times as the price of a more comfortable posture on the bike.

Position isn't the only thing to learn. You have to learn, again, to feel for your aerobic limit—and it feels different when you're speeding down the flats from the way it feels when you're climbing. Push a little too hard and you'll only last a mile or so. If you don't push hard enough, you'll know it when you finish . . . not even out of breath.

If you have no interest in competitive time trialing, these admonitions must sound grim. But even so, you should give yourself some occasional practice in this style of riding; here and there pick a flat three-mile stretch of road, put your nose down, and reach the end as quickly as possible. You'll develop the ability to ride at your maximum aerobic speed. In combination with interval training, time trial training will increase your maximum aerobic speed. And if riding at that speed is uncomfortable, riding just five percent slower can be comfortable. You can enjoy the pleasure of brisk, vigorous 20+ mph riding that feels downright relaxing. And you'll be fit enough to maintain that pace for hours. When you've reached that level, cycling will seem like an incredible reward.

7

Your Fitness Program

B y now you know something about the bike, pedaling and cadence, which is indeed a leg up on the majority of cyclists. What do you do now? More precisely, how do you specifically use your bike as a fitness tool?

Once you understand your bike, you should take a little time to understand your body. Though anecdotes in this book might suggest otherwise, it is essential that you practice prudence and restraint when starting an exercise program. Obviously, if you have diagnosed heart or circulatory problems, you should start out with one of the well-supervised programs available in most communities. Remember that the SCOR cyclists discussed in Chapter One started out that way. Today most of the SCOR cyclists have ridden single and double centuries.

If you have diabetes, asthma, or other conditions that would be affected by vigorous exercise, consult your doctor first. But keep in mind the success stories you've read about in this book. Doctors don't always encourage vigorous exercise. You have to take a certain amount of responsibility for your body.

Certainly don't start a cycling program if it will aggravate a foot or leg injury, though one real attraction of cycling is that many people who can't walk, can actually ride a bike. Furthermore, so gentle and forgiving is cycling that postoperative patients have had a great deal of success using cycling to regain strength and health.

If you are in reasonably good shape but have not exercised in 15 or 20 years, you should visit your doctor. Dr. Kenneth Cooper, founder of the aerobics movement, recommends the following for *inactive* people:

• Under age 30: Have a complete medical history and examination in the year before you get started.

• 30 to 35: The same, but do it within six months, and add a resting electrocardiogram (EKG).

• 35 to 40: All of the above, but within three months, and add a stress test.

• Over 40: All of the above, and a stress test. Plus a treadmill EKG if you have any risk factors: family history of high blood pressure, coronary problems or diabetes.

You might think that what Dr. Cooper recommends is conservative, and to a degree it is. Even the stress test has been subject to considerable criticism because it often fails to diagnose coronary narrowings in some individuals and registers false positives.

As important as what your doctor knows about you is what you know about yourself. Learn to take your pulse at rest at the wrist or temple. Count the number of beats for 15 seconds and multiply by four. You have your resting heartbeat. Make it a point to take your pulse on rising each morning.

As you will see, your pulse rate can tell you a lot. According to Tom Prehn, U.S. Olympic cyclist, "I can show you my training book. From the pulse rate you can see where I'm doing well and later when I'm starting to get sick. If my pulse is even just a beat off, it's noticeable."

In time you can be that sensitive to your pulse and what it tells you about your overall condition. You will know what food, drink and exercise does to your pulse. Properly observed, pulse can become a barometer and a guide.

Maximum and Training Heart Rates. As the accompanying formula suggests, you calculate your Maximum Heart Rate by subtracting your age from 220. (For the sake of accuracy women should use 226 rather than 220; the rest of the formula remains the same.) That is, if you are 40, doctors suggest that 180 is your MHR. And when training, you should raise your heart rate to no more than 70 to 85 percent of your MHR. That's called your Target Heart Rate and it's exactly that. Exercising at your THR will strengthen but not overstress your heart, lungs and legs.

Obviously, if you've been sedentary, you would start at the lower end of the scale, say 70 percent, and eventually increase your heart rate over weeks or months of training. If you experience signs of overexertion, such as dizziness and exhaustion, it is better to work at a lower heart rate.

TARGET HEART RATE

To determine your target (exercise) heart rate, complete the following formula:

220 − ____ = ____ Maximum Heart Rate   Resting Heart Rate ____
     Age

(MHR − RHR) .7 + RHR = ____ Target Heart Rate
(____ − ____) .7 + ____ = ____ THR

THR + 10 = ____
THR − 10 = ____

____ ←→ ____ Target Heart Rate Range
____ ←→ ____ THR for 6 Second Count

I've talked to many racers who regularly keep diaries. What kind of entries do they include? Jacques Boyer, the only American to have ridden in the Tour de France, keeps his entries short and simple. Weight, blood pressure, pulse, rate of ride (fast, medium, slow) and miles cycled. One reason competitive cyclists keep diaries is to become conscious of their cycling and training. According to Boyer, if he didn't keep a diary he'd forget how he trained and felt.

Some recreational cyclists just keep a mileage log with number of miles ridden and times, with totals for the months and year. Since you are using the bike as a fitness tool, you will likely want to do more. Before you begin your formal program, get a notebook and list your vital fitness functions: pulse, blood pressure, weight. Also list your fitness objectives. Do you want to lose weight, reduce stress, increase your lean body mass?

If you are to truly know and understand yourself and the effect exercise has on your body, you should also list in your diary other essential information about yourself including eating and snacking habits, alcohol and coffee consumption, and so on. Again, "Know thyself."

What to Put in Your Diary. When he was a world track sprinter, Canadian Gordon Singleton admitted that he took his diary everywhere, finding that an accurate record of his strengths and weaknesses prepared him for competition, particularly against Soviet riders.

Singleton used his diary "to record details such as how I felt during training or racing, what type of training I was doing (intervals, sprints or endurance), the number of miles per day." He also kept track of weather conditions because foul weather does influence the nature and quality of riding and training.

For the recreational cyclist, such detail is probably unnecessary, though whatever your level of accomplishment, it helps to keep track of your progress. Among headings you will probably want to include are:

- Resting heart rate (first thing in the morning).
- Number of miles ridden and in what gear.
- Length of ride—in time.
- Type of terrain.
- Exercise pulse rate.
- Type of riding.
- Weather conditions.

Many cyclists find it useful to note their general condition after the ride. Depending on how closely you want to monitor your performance, you might want to do the same thing. If you are equipped with cadence and heart monitors, you can keep a much more detailed record of your performance.

Whatever entries you include, don't let a diary complicate your life. If you don't like bookkeeping, keep the entries simple. Remember that a diary is a record and a motivator. It will keep you honest—and keep you going.

Almost anyone begins an exercise program wanting to lose weight. Fair enough, though you should probably take with a grain of salt the new weight and height charts published by insurance companies, which of late have been revised upwards as much as 13 pounds for men five-one to five-five, as well as lesser increases in the other categories. More significant is the percentage of lean body mass to fat. An average range for men and women is 8–20 percent and 18–30 percent, respectively. As part of your self-education, you can be measured, with caliper, at almost any YMCA, health club or at some job sites.

While not absolutely necessary, you might want to know your cholesterol level. If you've had a blood test of late, ask your doctor for it. Keep in mind that medical evidence suggests that cycling as little as 25 miles a week can reduce your overall cholesterol levels.

Try to get a handle on your calorie consumption. If I'm

any judge, I think most people are not particularly honest about the number of calories they consume—I know I'm not. ("I had a couple of beers.") Anything wrong with that human frailty? Perhaps not. Studies at Cornell University's Division of Nutritional Science have shown that exercise after eating uses up calories beyond the number used to directly perform the activity. According to David Levitsky, exercise is crucial in helping the body maintain a stable weight, even when the calorie consumption might fluctuate widely. For example, a gentle 20-minute walk within 45 minutes after a meal increases the number of calories the body burns as heat.

The moral of the story: You can still "lie" about your calories, just make sure you exercise after you eat. More importantly, be as conscious of what you eat as you are about exercise; you are bound to lose weight.

Your present condition will tell you how to go about starting your program. Keep in mind that most people get back into shape slowly. I'm assuming that it will take you a few weeks to get used to the bike and gearing. Don't consider that a waste of time. Consider it a safe way to recondition your body to gently put additional stresses on yourself. Don't worry about training effect until you have at least 4 to 5 weeks riding under your belt and can properly control your bike in all circumstances. As your steady state training increases, and your low gear spinning, your exercise tolerance will improve. Almost perceptibly, you will be adding minutes, yards and miles to your schedule. Your body will improve beneath you.

When you are sufficiently comfortable on your bike, take your THR from time to time, as a way of monitoring your progress, and note it in your diary. Within a month or so you should see your resting heart rate drop by at least a few beats a minute. If that is not the case, you might be exercising too hard.

At what intensity you should begin your exercise program and at what rate you should progress depends to some extent on your THR. For example, if you are between the age of 30 and 39, your THR range will be 130–160. If with your present level of conditioning you cannot operate easily in that range, your minimum program should be three 20-minute sessions a week at low resistance—in a low gear. Consider that your heart rate is a good guide to your overall aerobic capacity. Your immediate goal is to cycle comfortably within your THR range.

How to Begin. How you begin your cycling fitness program will depend on your age and general state of health. Here are some guidelines for the sedentary individual new to the sport.

Weeks 1 to 4. If you have been sedentary, see your doctor and get his or her approval. Start slowly. Cycle easily three times a week on a flat course for 20 minutes. Always start by "warming-up"—turning the pedals easily for 5 to 10 minutes to increase blood flow and prevent straining the muscles. "Cool down" by turning the pedals easily at the end of each exercise session to prevent muscle cramps and fatigue. Continue this program for a month, taking the time to understand the mechanics of your bike. Keep your bike in a middle gear to permit pedaling on flat terrain without exertion. At first, you'll want to increase your miles and time in the saddle quite rapidly. Resist the temptation—pushing too hard leads to injuries and discourages regular cycling.

As I said earlier, your first consideration should be to develop your cycling form, which includes your cadence and spin. So practice a brisk cadence and stay out of high gears.

Weeks 5 to 6. By the end of a month you will be ready to increase the *frequency, intensity,* and *duration* of exercise.

Expand the duration of your session to 30 minutes. At this point in your conditioning program time in the saddle is most important.

Week 7. By the end of the sixth week, you should add another day to your schedule, cycling for 30 minutes, four times a week.

Week 8. By the eighth week you should add one day of modest hill riding to your schedule. The hills should never be so steep as to require your lowest gear or anywhere near your maximum exertion. By the end of your second month you will be riding four times a week, 30 minutes a session, with one day of moderate hill riding.

Weeks 9 to 12. At the beginning of your third month you can increase the *duration* of your rides to 40–45 minutes. By this time you should be able to ride on almost any terrain, though it would still be sensible to balance your hill and flat riding.

Now you should be also ready to increase the *intensity* of your riding. You will have the necessary background miles to enable you to reach the lower end of your THR.

In your third month your emphasis should be on cycling *efficiently;* putting in more miles but not necessarily more time in the saddle.

Incorporate some modest *interval* training in your schedule, as defined elsewhere in this book.

Vary and adjust your program to meet your individual fitness and training goals. With this background, you should be ready for 30-to-40-mile rides. See Chapter Ten, Training for Long Rides. That will get you ready for your first century.

You might already be in fairly good shape from participating in other aerobic activities such as swimming or running or both. If you have been running or swimming three times a week for 30 minutes, your aerobic capacity should be such that you can operate comfortably in your

THR range. Nonetheless, if you're crossing over to cycling I would still recommend a breaking-in period of 3 to 4 weeks so you can get used to handling the bike and gears. There is no reason that you should not be able to cycle four times a week, thirty minutes a session, but your emphasis for the first few weeks should be on position and cadence. Coming from running you will likely be a "pusher" on the pedals—I was, and it will take some time to develop a brisk spin. Also, you will be tempted to engage your strong thigh muscles rather than all the muscles in your leg. I've ridden with some very strong runners who seem to take naturally to cycling. However, for the first couple of months I tend to stay clear of their wheels and handlebars because they have not yet developed a finesse of handling. But watch out when they get it.

The rate at which you add minutes to your basic exercise program will depend on how you progress. Just remember that your first fitness objective should be to improve your aerobic capacity, the ability of your lungs to handle oxygen.

Where you are doing your cycling will have some influence on the overall benefit. You might want to ride on relatively flat terrain during the first few weeks, then as your handling and balance become surer, add some modest hills to your ride. By the end of three weeks you should be able to increase the duration of your cycling to 30-minute sessions. After five or six weeks, you should add a day of cycling to your weekly calendar.

By this point in your beginner schedule you will be tempted to ride more miles in the same amount of time. That's a reasonable objective as long as you aren't pushing big gears and getting out of breath.

Now your attention should be to the quality of your workout, covering the mileage crisply and efficiently. Proper use of gearing should be second nature to you. Keep in mind that there is no absolute linear progression by which you should increase the frequency and duration of your cycling. Use your common sense. Because cycling is very easy, you might be tempted to increase your mileage quickly. Don't. Give yourself a couple of months to get the legs and lungs in shape.

Most researchers agree that you will improve your physical fitness if you exercise 30 minutes, four times a week. Other benefits, such as a reduction of body fat, will come if you increase the frequency of exercise. Later on, longer rides will take care of your body fat and specific weight training will increase your strength.

A TEN-WEEK SCHEDULE

In a week-to-week training schedule, these little tricks might fit in as follows:

Week 1 through Week 4:

SUNDAY—rest or easy (5- to 15-mile) ride.

MONDAY THROUGH FRIDAY—commute to and from work, shopping, or socializing once each day, not pushing hard (8 miles per day); on Wednesdays, take the long way home (12 miles at least).

SATURDAY—long (20- to 40-mile), easy ride.

Weeks 5 and 6:

SUNDAY—easy (5- to 15-mile) ride.

MONDAY THROUGH FRIDAY—mornings, easy commute (4 miles); Monday, Wednesday and Friday, easy commute home (4 miles); Tuesday and Thursday, 15-mile long way home; ride easily for first 6 miles, then 4 one-mile work intervals separated by one-mile rest intervals; 2 miles warm-down.

SATURDAY—long (30- to 50-mile), easy ride.

Weeks 7 and 8:

SUNDAY—easy (10- to 20-mile) ride.

MONDAY, WEDNESDAY AND FRIDAY—easy commute again; a few hard stoplight intervals on the way home.

TUESDAY—easy commute; long (20-mile) ride home with 3 or 4 long hill climbs and a few first-gear spinning binges in the middle.

THURSDAY—easy commute in; 15-mile ride home with 4 interval miles.

SATURDAY—long (40- to 80-mile) ride.

Weeks 9 and 10:

SUNDAY—easy (15- to 20-mile) ride.

MONDAY, WEDNESDAY AND FRIDAY—easy commute; stoplight intervals en route home.

TUESDAY, THURSDAY—easy commute to work; long (20-mile) ride home with 6 interval miles.

SATURDAY—long, relaxed (60- to 100-mile) ride.

There seems to be little debate among physiologists about the duration of aerobic exercise. To gain a significant training effect you should exercise for at least 20 minutes at 70 percent of heart rate capacity. And this should be done a minimum of three times a week. Of late, researchers have suggested that once you achieve a level of fitness, exercising a minimum of twice a week and perhaps only on weekends will give you a minimum level of fitness. Such a maintenance program might be a consideration later, once you reach an optimum level of fitness. However, if there were no more to cycling than a specific training effect, you could use it as you use situps. Unfortunately, you won't get the full physiological and psychological benefits from riding your bike on weekends.

If you are a new rider—new to cycling, and coming in with little or no conditioning—this training schedule will get you started and give you a rough idea of mileage for the first part of the season. If you follow these guidelines literally, you would increase your weekly mileage about ten percent, which is a reasonable increase. If you start out with some conditioning in another aerobic sport, such as running, you will likely be able to start with the June schedule. Remember that wherever you start, base mileage is more important than speed. Concentrate on cadence and spin.

If you are a beginner, you will want to ride every other day at first, until you become used to the bike. Within a week or so, you should be able to ride short distances five or six days a week. Figure on at least one rest day.

No matter what distance you ride, try not to ride at the same intensity two days in a row. A commonly accepted rule of thumb is that you alternate hard and easy days. For example, you shouldn't do interval-type training two days in a row. What you consider an easy day depends on what your hard workout is. A competitive cyclist might ride 140 miles one day and 70 miles the next. At your early stage of training your easy day will likely be a relaxed ride in a middle gear at a speed that doesn't significantly raise your pulse or make you breathe hard.

If you want to build your fitness program more closely around your Target Heart Rate (THR), you will want to keep careful record of that figure, most easily done in a diary. But don't be tempted to tie your program too closely to your THR because many events in your daily life impact your heart rate. Nonetheless, after a couple of months of regular cycling your resting rate should decrease and your training rate should increase.

If you follow this early-season schedule, cycling at high rpm in medium range gears for short time periods and at a regular frequency, what fitness benefits will you gain? Most important, you will be building up your base miles, so that later in your training you work harder and more efficiently. Almost imperceptibly, you will improve your cardiovascular condition; your high rpm will pump oxygen-laden blood through your body, opening up new capillaries, thus giving your muscles more capacity for work. You are training and strengthening your muscles so they will be ready for the longer and harder miles later on.

TABLE SIX

TRAINING SCHEDULE FOR NEW RIDERS

	Miles Per Day	Miles Per 5-Day Week	Miles on a Weekend
April	2–5	10–25	5–10
May	4–7	20–35	10–20
June	6–9	30–45	20–40
July	8–11	40–55	40–60

TABLE SEVEN

APPROXIMATE CALORIES EXPENDED DURING BICYCLING AT VARIOUS SPEEDS

Body Weight

Average Bicycle Speed	55 lbs. Calories per		110 lbs. Calories per		165 lbs. Calories per	
MPH	Min.	Hour	Min.	Hour	Min.	Hour
5.5	1.6	95	3.2	190	4.8	285
9.5	2.5	150	5.0	300	7.5	450
13.1	3.9	235	7.8	470	11.8	750

You should note some immediate benefits. Your resting pulse should drop and you should have more energy. You should lose weight or your lean body mass should increase. Remember it's not your total weight that's important but the percentage of lean body mass to fat. But if you keep your calorie intake constant, you will likely lose weight. The accompanying chart lists the calories you expend cycling at various rates per hour. Note that the speed of 13.1 miles an hour, well within the limits of a fast recreational rider, expends 750 calories an hour. Of course, the percent grade has a lot to do with how much energy you expend and how many calories you actually burn. More about that later.

If all goes well, after the initial struggle to increase aerobic capacity, you should start to find yourself paying more attention to other aspects of life, especially diet. In other words, your fitness program should begin with attention to miles, riding technique and target heart rate, but as you progress, you should consider your total body.

From that consideration will come total fitness.

8

Getting Better

A few years ago a West Coast charity bicycle ride for Muscular Dystrophy by Larry Christenson of the Philadelphia Phillies got a great deal of press—for the wrong reasons. Christenson fell off the bike when he failed to negotiate railroad tracks that ran diagonally across the road. He broke his collarbone and was out of action for a good part of the season.

At about the same time Ed Ott, then catching for the Pittsburgh Pirates, was riding to Florida for MD and fell at least three times while cycling through Baltimore. When I asked Ott about that, he said, "I'm not used to pedaling a bicycle with toe clips. I never gave a thought to getting my feet out of the toe clips. I was halfway to the pavement already."

When asked what was the most difficult part of cycling, Ott replied,

> Learning how to properly ride the bicycle. We had a representative from the Puch bicycle company along on the ride, and he was more or less our trainer. He taught us how to cycle. We were like country-boy bicyclists. We had no style whatsoever. I know for myself he really helped me with a lot of tips like keeping your knees in toward the bar [top tube].
>
> Another thing that really helped us a lot was

learning how to use the gears properly. The man from Puch was shouting out the gears to use as we rode. He might as well have said it in French, Spanish and German, because we had no idea what he was talking about until he gave us a chart explaining the gears.

Ott and the group of baseball and football players he was cycling with just assumed they could jump on their bikes and be competitive. After a number of incidents, accidents and falls, Ott realized that, although the bike is a fairly simple machine, the activity can become complex.

Whether you are coasting along or maintaining a brisk pace, cycling demands a lot. You are cycling on roads populated by cars and you have to be conscious of that fact at all times. If you are to cycle efficiently you must anticipate hills and select the right gears. You must balance and steer your bike, looking out for potholes and other constructions. And you must do all these things while moving at 15 to 20 miles an hour.

Good cycling is instinctive, a habit of action that is second nature. In this context I'm reminded of my favorite short story, "A Clean, Well-Lighted Place," by Ernest Hemingway. On the surface not a great deal happens in the story; it's the little things, the pauses, the gestures, the silence that give the narrative meaning.

The same is true of cycling in the hands of the artists. I recall watching a race in northern California. A lead group of about 20 had broken away from the rest of the pack and assumed the characteristic aerodynamic formation known as a peleton, trading off the pace in a kind of continuous give and take, give and go. Somehow a car had gotten onto the course but presented no hazard at first. Then the driver opened his car door seconds before the riders passed. The lead rider saw something, just in time. Perhaps he saw the man shift his weight over to the door or turn to see whether the coast was clear. At precisely the right time the lead rider turned smoothly and slightly to his left and the field followed, doing a snake dance around the open door and astonished motorist.

There is an inner game of cycling, an unconscious signaling of intention, and anticipation of another cyclist's need. Good cyclists don't make large movements. If they are moving around a pebble, they will miss it by millimeters. If an accomplished cyclist wants to pass on your left, he or she will likely move up and tap you on the shoulder, indicating he is coming by. If there is a turn to be made and you are following, look for a small finger indicating direction. This absence of obvious action is a function of style and form. The worst offense a competitive cyclist can commit is to be a sloppy bike handler. I recall watching a women's road race in Tuscon a few years ago. From my position in the press car I saw a group of about thirty riders go down. But somehow a few veteran riders tucked in the middle of the pack escaped that fate, even though cyclists all around them were spinning. I asked one experienced cyclist how she managed to stay up and she remarked "luck" and added, "Most people freeze in situations like that; they brake and grip the handlebars tight. I do just the opposite. I go with the flow and try to avoid any sudden movements."

Connie Carpenter, world cycling champion and one of the best female cyclists in the world, has said in an interview that the

> biggest problem most people have with bike handling is that they are not confident enough or relaxed enough to go with the flow. They panic and overreact, which is the worst thing you can do when you're handling your bike. For the women the biggest problem is they don't ride in large enough packs so that when they do get in a large pack, they don't know how to ride close to each other. If they bump handle-

bars or if someone swerves a bit, they overreact and that is where you get the majority of your accidents. Riding well in a pack is a matter of adapting and relaxing—your elbows should be bent, your shoulders and arms relaxed.

Riding in a group and practicing bumping handlebars and shoulders is good. It helps just to goof around on the bike more to become more relaxed. Many people are just too rigid on their bikes. Proper bike handling is simply a matter of riding more with more people and relaxing.

Greg LeMond, current World Professional Cycling Champion, has spoken about the inner game of cycling, about the ability of gifted athletes to anticipate. He recalled a hunting trip he took with three-time Tour de France winner Bernard Hinault. "A piece of shot ricocheted and hit my eye really hard. It put a hole in my eyelid. I'm saying, I just knew it was coming to me and I closed my eye, luckily!"

The ability to anticipate problems and to relax on a bike is the very essence of championship cycling form, which in itself implies a bond between rider and machine. The way you sit on a bike, the way your hands, feet and behind meet the bike, will dictate the quality of your cycling experience. This is all part of the etiquette, style and meaning of cycling.

Think of yourself as an Ernest Hemingway cyclist; your movements, gestures, and control of the bike are your aesthetics of cycling.

One of the real joys associated with cycling is to ride with friends, with people you can trust when you are moving at 25 mph. With group cycling, particularly among friends, there is a habit of cooperativeness and trust that is hard to match in any sport.

I have called cycling a very safe sport and it certainly is in the hands of good riders. But that does not mean that cyclists, including fast recreational riders, don't live on the edge of a certain kind of danger, like that associated with sky-diving, but more sensuous and controlled.

If you are sufficiently along in the sport, meaning you are as concerned about your equipment as about your body, you will likely be racing along on a bike that weighs less than thirty pounds. Chances are it could be closer to twenty. And your contact with the road might be the tread width of a one-inch tire. Therefore, you must trust your bike and those around it.

Once you have the background miles you will be drawn to a paceline like the wind to your back. The more confident you become, the closer you will ride your companion's wheel. The better you know that person, the more you will trust him or her.

One of my most pleasant bicycle rides is with two or three close friends on a 40-mile loop. I've cycled through more attractive landscape and on roads that are kinder to my tires. But this ride is special because we know it as we know each other.

Even if you forget the measurements, the pulse is always a part of the ride. We know each other's weaknesses and pounce on them like hungry kids whenever they show. I shake Len on that hill at the 23-mile mark. Randy leaves us in his wake at the west end of that tavern that sometimes calls when we don't remember home.

The semaphore of a tight-knit ride is written on the street. The finger that points idly to the road is not collecting air but pointing to a hole, a rut, a piece of glass.

The vertical bike that suddenly leans on its axis is not a vehicle out of control. There's a stone to be avoided. Yet the movement is not large. Blink and you could miss it.

On a gentle ride you run through the gears like a ratchet eating a chain. You take your landscape in bites.

You can feel when your cadence drops, so you find an extra tooth. Your hunger is always incremental. You nudge your shift lever, searching for the right cog. The chain drops on and your legs spin and sing.

Usually the process is orderly and predictable. When climbing a hill, you and your friends will find a lower gear. When descending, a higher one. The sound of the chain derailling gives away intention. On the downhill, if another's chain jumps the width of the cogs, you'll be chasing his wheel. On the way up, he might be chasing yours. But if on the climb he finds a higher gear, you might be in for a long afternoon.

Listen for the chain against the cage. Watch his hand fidgeting on the downtube. Watch him rise out of the saddle like a beginning racer. He is ready to play.

You know when a serious cyclist is ready for business. At the start of the ride the cyclist yawns uninterestedly on the tops of the bars. His feet are lazily in the toe clips. The straps are not tight; they hang down like clotheslines.

But by mile five, the nose is closer to the handlebars and the feet are tucked tightly into the pedals. Now the ride begins.

To become a better cyclist means getting good at the little things. Chances are that when you started, you started cycling "heavy," which has nothing to do with your weight. It refers to the way you sit on the bike and how you handle yourself in a crowd of cyclists.

With practice and concentration you can ride light and confident, as if your fingers and brain are doing all the work.

9

Dressing Right

T hree years ago I was cycling with two friends from Allentown, Pennsylvania, to Rhode Island for a cycling convention. When the three of us started our journey, the sun was hot and the skies clear. By the time we reached the Blue Mountains twenty miles north of Allentown, a cold front had swept in. The temperature dropped thirty degrees in a matter of minutes and the rains came and the winds howled. Almost before we had time to put on our rain parkas, we were chilled. My hands were so cold I couldn't operate my brake or shift gears. I felt a lowering of my body temperature and we wisely stopped for food and coffee until the storm had passed.

That ride was in late June. Thank goodness for our wool cycling jerseys that soaked up much of the rain, though by the time we passed through Connecticut those jerseys seemed too heavy.

Such swings in temperature and climate are not uncommon anywhere in the country and indicate that cycling clothes must be very functional. What you wear has a direct relationship with how you perform on a bike. In this chapter I'm concerned about function rather than fashion, though you will hear enough about the latter. Briefly then, if you want to be a tight, neat, aerodynamic unit on your bike it hardly makes sense to wear your pyjamas.

Jerseys. Generally speaking, cycling clothes have to perform well under many conditions. You want a jersey to keep you cool when the weather's hot, hot when it's cool, dry when it's wet. You want a jersey that feels good, feels light—and all for a low price.

You might not think that you will do the type of riding that will make demands on a jersey. Consider if you go out for an early morning ride in the summer. You are into your third month of training so you can do 50–60 miles with no difficulty. If you start at sunrise with the temperature sixty degrees Fahrenheit, you will also have to deal with the wind chill that develops as you ride at 15 mph. Depending on your clothing, you could be cold. What do you do, what do you wear? This is a question that should concern every cyclist who rides for exercise because if you're not comfortable you will not get the most benefits from cycling.

Cycling jerseys, probably your most important item of clothing because they cover the greatest body area, come in a wide selection of fabric. Gone are the days when the only choice on the market was a European brand with all sorts of weird writing (sponsors' names) across the front and back. Today jerseys come in wool, cotton, polyester, polypropylene, nylon and acrylic fibers. You can still get the weird writing, but only if you choose.

Is there one type of fabric that is best suited for cycling? No. The choice of a cycling jersey, like any article of clothing, is very subjective, but here are some guidelines.

Bicycling magazine's Product Testing arm has examined and tested under actual riding conditions 38 jerseys currently on the market. While not including all the available jerseys, this was a representative sampling. The jerseys were used during a variety of weather and climate conditions generally found during spring and summer in the eastern part of the U.S.

The twelve test riders, including myself, arrived at no absolute consensus. Preferences and riding styles played a large role. However, the wool jerseys and the wool blends were the favorite, due in part to thermal comfort. Wool provides warmth when the weather is cool and dryness when it is wet. Even on hot days wool handled perspiration better than the polypropylene jerseys. Overall, the testers thought that wool is the best choice when you have one jersey that has to satisfy a number of cycling conditions.

You will find, as our testers did, that wool and acrylic blends are very close to pure wool in feel and performance, yet do not weigh as much. The cotton jerseys, which felt good against the skin on dry, sunny days, tended to soak up water and sag, especially at the hem and pockets in the back. The cotton/polyester jerseys we examined were similar to the pure cotton samples but like the former would not be recommended for cold weather.

One trend in cycling wear is toward polypropylene jerseys which are lightweight and stretchy, wrapping the body like a stocking. Though wool seemed a little superior on hot, dry days, polypropylene would not absorb as much moisture in the rain and therefore would not be as heavy as wool.

We found the acrylic jerseys to be comfortable with the right amount of stretch. Thermal comfort was adequate in a variety of cycling conditions and climates. The nylon/lycra jerseys will give you the sleek look of a bike racer but with a significant loss of thermal insulation for cool weather cycling.

Before buying a jersey, think about construction as well as use. Turn the jersey inside out and check the seams for workmanship signaled by neat stitches and tight seams.

You might want to consider three pockets rather than two as the load you carry—food, spares, etc.—will hang more evenly.

Since you are often stretched out on a bike, the jersey should not ride up; allow for it to extend about eight inches below your waist. When you are standing straight the jersey should reach the middle of your buttock. A jersey that is too small is very uncomfortable because it exposes the lower part of your back to the sun and air.

So what jersey should you buy? Consider your pocketbook, your riding style, and the range of weathers you will be cycling in. Wool has many advantages but the cost is a little higher than the other fabrics—$36 to $49 at retail. The cotton/polyester, polypropylene, and acrylic jerseys start closer to $20. So price is a consideration.

Keep in mind that a wool jersey will likely function better under a variety of weather conditions, though most cyclists tend to switch to a lighter fabric when the weather gets really warm. By all means put insulating value and moisture control high on your list of criteria. If a jersey doesn't keep you warm and soak up moisture without feeling like a rag, saving a few dollars is little consolation.

As engineer David Sellers concluded in his study of jerseys,

> Keeping cool is a matter of wearing thinner jerseys with a porous knit to allow body moisture to pass through (whether by wicking or absorption), and a fit just loose enough to permit some air to circulate across the skin, promoting convection cooling. Keeping warm dictates a thicker, bulky, tightly knit jersey with a comfortable tight fit to discourage convection cooling. Of course, layering is always a good option to fall back on; one combination that seems to work well is to wear a fairly open wicking fabric next to the skin, with a good quality fabric over it.

Buying a jersey is a very personal decision, as is the purchase of any piece of clothing. You can buy jerseys through the mail, though I recommend you go to a bike shop that will actually let you try on the product. I've been on mass cycling rides consisting of up to 10,000 cyclists. Of the people in cycling clothes, many appear to be wearing jerseys that are too small. Accordingly, when they stretch out on the handlebars, their backs are exposed. Whether this is due to a poor purchase in the first place or incorrect washing, there's no way to tell. My point here is for you to make sure the jersey fits you in the first place, then you care for the fabric properly.

For the clothing-conscious cyclist or the cyclist who rides all year, there is a veritable wardrobe to choose from. The jerseys discussed above are all short-sleeve, but you can find most of these fabrics in long-sleeve versions. You can also buy rainsuits, windbreakers, cool weather tights and even booties to keep your feet warm.

You will certainly want full-length cycling clothes if you intend to be cycling in the spring and autumn when the wind chill significantly lowers the temperature. Keep in mind that many amateur and professional riders don't get out of their long wear until the outside temperature reaches sixty degrees.

You can build up your wardrobe as your cycling develops. You might want a windbreaker (with holes for air circulation) for spring and autumn rides. Or you might want raingear if you intend to ride when it's wet. These items you can add when appropriate.

When choosing your cycling clothing, think about function as much as fashion. Fortunately these days, you can get both at a good price. Consider the type, frequency and intensity of your cycling, as well as your location.

If you are an April to September recreational cyclist, you can likely get away with purchasing a minimum of two short-sleeve cycling jerseys and two pairs of shorts. But if you cycle with greater intensity and frequency, if your cycling includes intervals and long rides in all types of weather, you will need a few more jerseys, including at least one with long sleeves.

Hygiene is an important consideration and your type of riding will dictate how often you can use a jersey. Good health habits should govern your decisions.

If you want to cycle all year, you will want to invest in a fuller wardrobe, including cool weather tights, windbreaker and rainsuit. Cyclists who ride in extremely cold weather often wear thick ski gloves and boots to fit over cycling shoes.

The point is there is a rich array of cycling clothing to satisfy your needs. Let economics and good sense be your guide. If you plan to cycle moderately—say three times a week, during the warmer weather—you might be able to get by with one pair of shorts and a jersey. If you do encounter some unseasonably low temperatures, you can always wear a long-sleeve garment under your cycling jersey, though you really shouldn't cycle in shorts if the weather gets much below sixty degrees Fahrenheit. The wind chill can cool off your knees very quickly.

Cycling Shorts. These come in a variety of fabrics from wool to polypropylene and in enough daring colors to make the European cycling community wince.

Since you wear cycling shorts more for comfort than insulating effect, though that obviously is a consideration when the weather is cool, I'll concentrate on the former consideration. The vast majority of recreational cyclists don't wear cycling shorts and probably don't need to. If you're coasting along at five to six miles an hour once or twice a week you are certainly getting out in the air but not getting much exercise. For those people, cycling shorts are not necessary.

But as soon as you increase your rpms and spend a little

more time on a bike, you will find that cutoffs chafe and cause blisters. While writing this book I decided to hop on my Monarch exercise bike and spin for an hour. My cycling shorts and touring shoes were upstairs and that was too much bother so I cycled for an hour in running shorts and tennis shoes. The next day I had a large blister on the inside of my thigh from the chafing.

Cycling shorts, whether they are made of wool or cotton, possess a number of important features. They fit snugly, coming well down on the thigh, and don't creep up. They also contain a chamois, a lining which serves as padding for the crotch area. With no seams, cycling shorts do not irritate the skin. For $20 you cannot make a better investment in comfort.

Shoes. I have written about the biomechanics of cycling, which is the study of the interaction between rider and machine. The body meets the bike at three points—pedal, saddle, and handlebars, and it's important that this "meeting" be as comfortable as possible. New cyclists have problems in precisely these areas because they tend to absorb too much road shock through the bike—especially through their feet.

For a long while little attention was paid to cycling shoes. Over the years, however, there has been a proliferation of information on running shoes, and extensive tests have been made by the Biomechanics Lab at Pennsylvania State University. Most people assume they can cycle in tennis shoes, which for the short-distance cyclist is not a bad decision. But if you want maximum performance from your bike and if you want to be truly one with your machine, you have to use cycling shoes and toe straps. And probably cleats.

A few years ago I would go to a ride and see hundreds of fancy custom bikes ridden by cyclists in tennis shoes. While that has changed somewhat, there is still a tendency on the part of beginners and recreational cyclists to scorn cycling shoes as apparatus for the professional.

I frequently attend large touring rides for charity, which usually mean a cycling leg of 70 to 100 miles in a day. The good people who have collected pledges for each mile to be ridden usually arrive with a decent bike but rarely with decent shoes. I've given belated advice to dozens of riders whose feet ached by mile ten.

The reason is simple. Tennis shoes or the familiar jogging shoes don't have a stiff enough shank to absorb all the stresses which radiate out from the pedal to various parts of the foot. A stiff-soled cycling shoe absorbs most of the stresses and prevents them from reaching your feet.

Touring shoes are a compromise. Shoes such as Bata, Detto Pietro, Avocet, Le Coq Sportif, Puma, Sedi, Nike and others have a fairly stiff shank that enables you to push down on the pedals without feeling the stresses on your feet, though there are great differences among brands. With most touring shoes you can get off the bike and walk around, though not for long distances.

Most people who want the bike to fit them like a glove insist on cycling shoes with cleats, a metal attachment that locks your foot in position on the pedals so that there is neither lateral nor fore and aft movement. With cleats your foot won't move around on the pedals. In turn, you can pedal faster and maintain good form without putting in any extra effort.

I might as well get the objections out of the way first. You might feel that being locked into the pedal by toe clips, straps and cleats is dangerous. Actually, it isn't. First of all you are never really locked into the pedals. The cleat has a groove that slides down over the pedal cage and secures the foot. Tightening the toe strap just makes your foot more snug on the pedal. *No matter how tight you are cleated into your pedals, in an emergency you can always pull your feet out*.

Adding toe clips to your bike is an early step to help improve your cadence and form on the bike. Adding cleats is a second step. Compared to a few years ago there are dozens of brands of cleated shoes available, including Adidas, Avocet, Sedi, Detto Pietro, Duegi and Puma.

I'd recommend that you shop around for shoes in your area bike shops. A good pair of shoes will cost you $40 and up and last for years. As you would with any shoe, try on the cycling shoe first and make sure it fits. European models tend to be narrow, though that is changing, particularly with the competition from American manufacturers. And European sizes are different, so consult the comparison charts carefully before you buy. No matter what the salesperson says, fit is still the most important consideration.

The best cycling shoe has a leather upper and holds the foot firmly and allows it to breathe. It also conforms to the shape of the foot. Most have small holes in the toe box for that reason. Keep in mind that cycling shoes are still a specialty item, that they are available only through the cycling distribution system. While that might well keep prices a little high, it does ensure that you will not be as plagued by imitations as we are with running shoes.

There is no *best* cycling shoe. Recently Mitchell L. Feingold, Doctor of Podiatry, performed lab tests on 27 pairs of cleated shoes. Twenty-three different items were evaluated on each shoe. He notes that which shoe is best for you depends on your foot structure and how much you are willing to pay.

With the help of the Department of Mechanical Engineering at San Diego State University, Feingold measured the sole stiffness of each pair of cycling shoes. The test indicated that the Duegi Supercompetizione was the stiffest and the Le Coq Sportif Hinault Competition was the most flexible. So what does all this mean?

It depends. If you are planning to engage in a heavy race schedule, you will likely choose the Duegi over the

Le Coq model. If you plan some moderately hard riding on the order we have discussed, your choice probably won't make a lot of difference. Similarly, the test indicated that at 242 grams the Duegi was the lightest shoe while at 394 grams the Diamont Sprint was the heaviest. Will 152 grams make a lot of difference to the fast recreational rider? Probably not.

The same test indicated that the combined sole and cleat thickness of the Diadora Mondial was 1 cm, while the thickness of the Diamont Sprint was 2.2 cm. Is this significant? Perhaps, particularly for a cyclist who wants extra padding on his feet.

Based on his laboratory tests, Dr. Feingold recommends that you "choose a shoe that has a reasonably stiff sole, a cleat that has a deep and narrow slot which grips the pedal cage firmly and a sole that is flat at the contact point with the pedal so as not to allow the shoe to rock." Above all, Feingold suggests you buy a shoe that fits and allows you to place your foot in the right position on the pedal. He also recommends a shoe with enough ventilation holes in the upper and soles for the passage of excess moisture.

A change from tennis or jogging shoes to *any kind* of cycling shoe will bring increased comfort and improve your pedaling. You will not feel the pedal cage through your shoes, with the exception of some of the touring shoes that are very flexible and not designed for rides over 20 to 30 miles.

You might consider that the benefit of being able to walk around in touring shoes outweighs the disadvantages (flexible sole and movement of foot on the pedal). If so, purchase a shoe with the stiffest sole you can find and get on with your cycling.

If you want to move to the next level in bike fit and your own performance, buy a cycling shoe that will accept cleats. Most shoes available in the U.S. have adjustable cleats that are already attached to the shoes. These cleats can be moved forward, backward or rotated until you find the best position. To find that position you should, with the help of a friend, sit on your bike and experiment. When you've found the right position, secure the cleats in place by bolts, nails or screws.

Some shoes found in bike shops don't come with cleats; they have to be purchased separately which sometimes is an advantage. You might want a deeper cleat than normally offered, but whatever you choose make sure the shape of the cleat conforms to the sole of the shoe. If you want some help with your cleats, enlist the aid of a cycling friend. Or go to your local bike shop. When I'm putting on a new set of cleats I always go to my local bike shop where I have the benefit of an expert eye and opinion to make sure that my cleat placement conforms to my position on the bike.

But, whoever helps you with your cleats, be fussy about placement. As you now know, the axle of the pedal should lie directly under the ball of the foot. If the cleat puts your foot too far back on the pedal, the toe muscles will be strained and the heel of the shoe will tend to come off the foot. If your foot is too far forward, the shoe will push up into your arch and you won't be able to fully engage your calf muscles.

Make sure that your toe points straight forward on the pedal, unless your physiology demands otherwise. The key consideration is to keep joint movement to a minimum. I have ridden with cycling shoes for a few days so the pedal makes an indentation on the sole of the shoe, permitting more accurate marking and placement of cleats. If you are going to do the same thing, be sure that your toe clips are not too large or your feet are not moving around on the pedal. That could give you a false reading.

When you are ready to actually put the cleats on your cycling shoes, get help from a friend or a bike shop. Your "riding marks" will give you a pretty good idea of placement, but you should be exact. The marks should be made on the soles while you are seated on the bike. You might want to tack the cleats in place and ride for a few miles to check for comfort and position. You should leave about a quarter of an inch between your toe and the toe clip.

You will find that by using cycling shoes, cleats and toe clips you will truly be a part of the bike. Important to your training program, you will naturally increase your rpm and be more conscious of gearing. You will pull up on the toe straps as you get to the bottom—dead center—of your pedaling cycle. You will be a more efficient cyclist and the time you devote to exercise will be better spent.

This will take practice and work. Everyone can push down on the pedals, that's a normal range of motion. But not everyone can pull up on the pedals. When you turn the pedals you circumscribe an arc of perhaps 340 mm (two 170-mm crank lengths) so your feet stay in a very tight circle. When you reach the bottom of the pedal stroke the clips and cleats allow you to complete the circle, pulling up for power and fuller leg involvement—and engagement of the quadriceps.

There is still some debate about how much power pulling up on the straps actually delivers to the pedals. To a certain extent I consider that beside the point. I am talking about improving your cycling technique and your position on the bike. For the bicycle to be truly a fitness tool, a responsive machine beneath you, it has to be an extension of you. Think of the use of toe straps and cleats not as confinement but as liberation. The bike now belongs to you. Instead of jumping on your bike in sloppy fashion in boots and jeans, you've slipped into it as you would a good suit. Instead of cranking along in high gear, tiring quickly, you match your gearing to the strength of your legs and heart. Instead of simply pushing down on the pedals, you pull up, in perfect control of your progression. You don't go to pieces when you are approaching a stop sign or red light. You understand that as part of the ritual. You anticipate, slow down, loosen one toe strap and be ready in case you have to stop.

I have written about form at some length. The height of your saddle, the length of your cranks, top tube and stem will dictate what kind of ride you will have. If your saddle is too high, you will be reaching for the pedals, moving your hips too much. If your stem or top tube is too long, you will be extending yourself too far. You want neither of these conditions. Rather you want to be a tight unit over the bike, you want your center of gravity to be concentric.

In a way a good cyclist is like a good boxer who keeps his hands close to his face and body for protection, and throws short punches of less than 18 inches. Sure of where his feet are at all times, the boxer is tucked in tight and very efficient. To swing wild would be sloppy.

A bike rider also occupies a very narrow, though moving space. Most of his weight is over the pedals which turn in a small 340-mm arc. With toe clips, straps and cleats, the arc is always the same. And the plane is similar to the movement of wheels, axles and the bike itself. With knees and elbows in and the cycling clothing providing a shell, the rider works efficiently within a narrow, closely defined space. To veer out of that space would be inefficient and sloppy.

To be in the uniform of the day on a bike that fits and having the legs that will carry you through is, in the words of Jacques Boyer, who finished 12th in the 1983 Tour de France, "Exhilaration, health."

10

Training for Long Rides

A couple of years ago I decided to cycle from Allentown, Pennsylvania, to Dayton, Ohio, to attend a cycling convention. As I'm suggesting in this book, I put in a lot of early base mileage. I commuted to work as often as I could and took longer rides on Saturdays and Sundays. I was on a good schedule for a traditional September century, but my ride to Dayton was in June and I felt the paucity of my training after riding hard for a day in the Pennsylvania hills. I got by, but it didn't have to be that way. I should have known better. I did, but I thought I could cheat a little on early-season training. No way.

With an adequate base, almost anyone can ride a century in 10 to 12 hours. Like a running marathon, a bicycle century will sooner or later call you. In September of each year the League of American Wheelmen, the oldest cycling organization in the country, conducts a century month, awarding patches for all those who test the distance. The League also offers patches for doing 25 miles in 3 hours, 50 in 6 hours, a metric century (100 km or 62 miles) in 7.5 hours, and a century in 12 hours (or less). If you want to get your hands on these patches—particularly for the century—you should begin early. And no matter what your level of proficiency early in the season, with the right training you can complete a century in September—without pain. Consider some people who have.

Dennis M. Tapp, of Portland, Oregon, wounded in an armed robbery, suffered spinal cord, liver and kidney damage. Then a myocardial infarction—heart attack. He could hardly walk. On the advice of his cardiologist, he started riding a stationary bike, giving it up because it was boring. So he purchased a bicycle, nothing fancy—a 42-pound special from Penney's. He tells me, "I must have looked like a joke on that bicycle because I could not ride well, and I had to be sure not to stop and lean on my right leg (because of the heavier paralysis)."

Fifteen years later Mr. Tapp has ridden a century, cycled across America, and to Alaska. He is capable of cycling 50 to 100 miles a day.

"Who knows," he says rather whimsically, "maybe one of these days I might be able to walk normal again (or even run)."

To say anyone can ride and profit from regular cycling is an understatement and fact; everyone can. Cycling is so forgiving, in the biomechanical sense, that you can do as little as turn the pedals at first and by season's end you can be riding a century. Such a distance is within the range of anyone who prepares.

You could probably continue on the early-season schedule outlined in this book and maintain a reasonable level of fitness. But I don't know anyone who doesn't take a certain amount of pleasure in being able to increase his or her mileage. Furthermore, as you have seen in the success stories, it is very important to have goals and objectives which give you something to work for. You might not put a century on your calendar, but put something on you can work toward, even if it's no more than a 25-mile ride.

You will find that during the early part of your training your time will probably improve rather quickly. On the other hand, once you get to your optimum and comfortable speed—say 15 mph—improvements will come more slowly. Don't worry about that as there will be other improvements that will not be so noticeable, such as the way you position yourself on the bike. With practice you will learn to relax more on a bike and arrive at your destination less fatigued.

By all means keep an account of your mileage, if only to keep yourself honest. If you'd like a free copy of a mileage log, send a postcard to me at *Bicycling* magazine. The address can be found in the Appendix.

TRAINING FOR THE CENTURY

Before he became an Olympic-caliber racer cycling more than 300 miles a week, Tom Prehn decided to ride a century. He notes that the

> distance sounded immense, forbidding, bordering on the limits of human endurance. Surely if I could do it, I would prove something—my macho, my strength, call it what you want, the accomplishment would make me feel like Superman.
>
> As it turned out, for me, the Mt. Hamilton Challenge was well named. It was more than the required 100 miles, 130 to be exact, and involved about 4,000 feet of climbing. Was I ready for it?
>
> Not very. On that unforgettable day a friend to whom I'm forever grateful helped and encouraged me through the last 70 miles when my magnificent machine became an instrument of torture. Some invisible string, stretched from his big form in front of me, pulled me through it. Without him I certainly would have quit.

Of course, afterward I was elated. I'd done it. A hundred miles, unbelievable! I was also shattered. I couldn't walk. The day following the ride Superman stayed in bed, stiff, miserable and sore.

Before Prehn became a brilliant Olympic racer, he shared some similarities with recreational cyclists who, after putting in a few basic trips decided to ride a century— and a tough century at that. It's the equivalent of running 15 to 20 miles a week and then participating in a marathon. The governing words here are prudence and caution; don't be tempted to ride a century before you are ready. For that matter, don't be tempted to undertake any long ride. Progress at your pace and speed and watch out for the "hotdogs."

You will perform much better in your long ride if your training is gradual and over at least a three-month period. Most new cyclists will be able to complete a century after a 12-week program. Some cyclists, depending on their level of fitness and physical state, will need more time. Treat the following schedule as a very rough guide that you should adapt to meet your own needs.

My first rule of thumb is to make sure you have the base miles in. This could mean very short rides and very little mileage, but get on your bike early in the season (or stay on with an exercise bike). Conditioning your body is more important than conditioning your legs in the early part of the season.

Weeks 1–2. Try and get on your bike every day even if your rides are only 2 to 3 miles. Don't even bother with the larger gears as this period is for high rpms and low gears. Cycle a minimum of 30 miles a week and by the end of the second week you should be riding 10 miles without stopping.

Weeks 3–6. During this period you should increase your total weekly mileage from about 30 to 80 or 90. Start to think about where you ride and how you ride. As you spend more time on the road, try and divide your schedule into hard and easy days, which refers to the pace of the ride as well as terrain.

Let your daily schedule dictate your training schedule. Most people seem to have a little more time on weekends than during the week and that is probably the time for longer rides. During weeks three and four you still want to concentrate on just putting in the miles on relatively flat terrain which will give you the opportunity to get used to your gearing and improve your cadence to the 80–90 rpm range.

By the fifth week, you should be ready to balance hard and easy training days. For example, you might want to take a long ride of 20 to 30 miles nonstop on a Sunday at a brisk pace. On Tuesdays, a *hard* day of training, your emphasis should be on time rather than distance. Cycle for a minimum of 30 minutes at a hard, fast cadence, including hills as your condition permits. This kind of training will help improve your overall strength and aerobic conditioning. On this schedule, Wednesday will be a light day, with a gentle 5-to-10-mile ride and Thursday a hard training day.

Your goal during this period is to increase your weekly mileage to about 80 or 90. If you are going on a long ride, there is no shortcut in this area. You are also improving your strength and aerobic conditioning. But remember that no one knows your body better than you do. Listen to it. Check and record your pulse, especially after your hard days. And monitor your weight. If you don't feel like cycling long or hard on a particular day, don't do it; your body is telling you something. And don't feel compelled to follow any of this advice literally. There's no way around the fact that, if you want to do a century, you should be cycling 4 to 5 hours a week. How you do it is another matter. Don't get so caught up in a training regimen that you lose your interest in the sport. And don't feel guilty if you skip a day—it's probably good for you.

Weeks 7–10. You should be building on the previous 6 weeks' effort by staying with the same hard and easy routine and by increasing your weekly mileage from 80 to 140. Longer rides are very important at this stage so try and schedule one for Sunday and one in the middle of the week. By now you should be ready to cycle 50 miles on a Sunday (or a Saturday, if it's more convenient). Also try to get in a 30-to-40-mile drive during the week. I have noticed in my own training that the mid-week ride makes a great difference when I'm riding a century. You can get by on a schedule that just includes a long weekend ride, but try to find time during the week.

Weeks 11–12. This is the time to fine-tune your training. Plan to cycle around 140 miles each week. As important as the total mileage is your doing two long rides back-to-back, preferably on a Saturday and a Sunday. During week 11, plan two 40-mile rides, week 12, two 50-mile rides. On your hard days add some interval training. Very simply, interval training is going as hard as you can for a short distance, until you are functioning anaerobically (without oxygen). You want to get your heart rate up to 70–85 percent of maximum. Nothing complicated about this. Just pick a landmark a short distance away and pedal as fast as you can toward it. Do that a few times during a work-out. Many cyclists I know use telephone poles, which seem to appear with a disturbing frequency.

If you have followed this training schedule, however loosely, you will have ridden a little less than 1,000 miles, which is ample preparation for a century ride. During the week of the ride, cycle no more than 10 miles on the two days before the event, which will likely be on a Saturday or Sunday. With the preparation you've done, the ride should be a piece of cake. More later on how to ride a century.

If you have a reasonably high level of fitness and substantial base mileage (say, 100 miles a week), you can probably train for a century in a little over a month by improving the quality of your training.

For the three weeks prior to a century you should increase your total mileage to 150, which should include two long (40–50 miles) rides a week. Build on the training you have already been doing, but make sure you follow the easy and hard regimen. In the third week add some intervals to your training. Ease off your training during the fourth week. Ride every day but at a more relaxed pace.

It's one thing training for a century, another riding it, for even some of the best-trained and most knowledgeable cyclists sometimes forget what they have learned on the morning of the century and think they are in a race. They are not. Nor are you.

Chances are, if you join a local club for a formal century ride you will be joined by dozens of other cyclists. Some large clubs bring out hundreds. While you can certainly ride a century on your own—many people do—the thrill of riding with other cyclists is hard to match. After all, a century ride is a social and family activity.

On the other hand, there are always a few who bolt from the pack and dash for the finish line. Unless you are in very good shape, say good-bye to them. Cardinal rule number one: Ride a century at your own pace. There are only winners in this game.

TRAINING FOR TOURING

If you plan to tour with cycling bags and the like, you could be carrying around 30 to 40 pounds of luggage. Thus, you won't be as interested in going fast as in cycling long distances. Furthermore, handling a loaded bike demands different techniques and certainly calls for more upper body strength.

Rather than planning for a century you might plan to cycle across your state or from one city to another or even across country. If you'd like to be more of a long-distance tourist, don't worry about not getting fit. A few years ago a Ball State research group tested a group of forty cyclists before and after a 4,000-mile cross-country cycling trip which lasted about five weeks. Average mileage: 120 miles a day, which is well within the limits of a moderately trained cyclist. The research found that the cyclists decreased their heart rates from an average of 87 to 57 beats per minute and decreased their average exercise heart rate from 152 to 117 beats per minute. All girth measurements decreased.

Many cyclists build their season around a solo or group tour (or tours) with emphasis on cycling long, slow distances. The training requirements for this kind of cycling are a little different from fast recreational riding, not in total miles but in types of riding and training.

Whether you are planning to ride a century with the local cycling club in September or take a month-long cross-America trip, you will still need the base mileage. However, after you've gotten your sea legs, and your bottom, back and wrists are used to the bike, your emphasis should be on long steady distance (LSD) training rather than intervals. At least once a week you will still want to begin with one day of hard, nonstop riding, 10 miles at first, then 40 miles during your third month of training.

You will still want to ride 40 to 50 miles twice a week and probably participate in at least one century before a long, multi-day tour. You should also spend a lot of time in the hills, seeking them out particularly when you are feeling good. When I am training for a long tour (Pennsylvania to Rhode Island or Ohio), I devote at least two days a week to hill climbing and usually consider them a "hard" workout. I often ride up and down the steepest hill I can find until I can't do it anymore.

If you are planning a long tour with packs you should make sure your upper body is strong enough to handle a loaded bike. The best way to do this is with weights, a subject I'll be discussing a little later. You should also take trial runs with your loaded bike so you get a feel for handling. With 30 to 40 extra pounds your bike will take longer to stop and the feel will be much different.

Cycling touring is a rich activity within the sport of cycling that offers a pleasant, noncompetitive way to stay fit. In the Appendix you will find a list of group tour outfits that offer thousands of touring possibilities all over the world. But, depending on your interests and inclinations, you might want to pick your own way across a state or the country or travel with the family and friends. Whatever approach you choose, you will become fitter in the process.

If you are not training for specific goals such as amateur or club races or improving your times in particular distances, bicycle touring is a very pleasant way to stay fit. Through the contacts in the Appendix you can find the touring club closest to you.

INTERVAL TRAINING

Many athletes have discovered that interval training helps improve their cardiovascular conditioning with minimum investment in time. In cycling, interval training will improve your pace and your performance in the hills.

Don't even consider engaging in interval training until you have at least a month's riding—three to four hundred miles—under your belt. To do so on less mileage will invite knee and tendon problems. Consider that an absolute rule.

When you are ready for an interval workout, find yourself a flat road. Warm up in a low gear for about 20 minutes. There is no set length or intensity for intervals so base your program on your conditions. Try to include in your workout four work periods of five minutes' duration followed by a three- or four-minute rest period, then warm down in a low gear for 20 minutes.

Your aim in interval training is to bring your training heart rate up to about 80 percent of maximum, based on the formula provided earlier. Just because you are supposed to work hard during interval training, don't be lured into using a high gear. Remember that you still want your pedal cadence to be high, actually 20 to 30 rpms higher than your normal cadence. So choose your gear carefully.

Don't get off the bike during your rest period; keep pedaling in a low gear. And don't do intervals more than twice a week. Vary the length and intensity of them, depending on how you feel. If you've had a long ride on a Sunday you might not feel like working quite so hard. On such occasions, perform more interval repetitions but not at such intensity.

Intervals are a very useful and personal form of training, of getting better quickly. But to gain maximum benefit from this tool, you must understand your body. Make sure you don't jump into interval work without sufficient background mileage and that you don't overdo a good thing. Keep close watch on your pulse, your weight, and your general well-being.

One important aid in your training and commitment to cycling is to join a touring or racing club. There are hundreds of cycling clubs in the country and one within reasonable distance of where you live. Check with your local bike club. If you want to join a touring club, contact the League of American Wheelmen, a racing club, or contact the United States Cycling Federation. Addresses are listed in the Appendix.

Note that many clubs offer both touring and racing opportunities. Much club riding can be called fast recreational riding, a fine regimen for the fitness-minded, but if you want to proceed to the next step—racing—by all means join the United States Cycling Federation and acquire an amateur racing license. The USCF offers age categories for both sexes and hundreds of races in which you can get your feet wet. Bike racing is a physical and intellectual challenge for those with a competitive spirit. Note that the training schedules outlined in this book would serve as a good grounding for readers interested in racing, although you should have at least a minimum of 1,000 base miles and considerable group and club riding experience before you become a beginner (Category 4) racer.

11

Your Championship Form

F rom good position on a bike comes good form and technique. And fitness. As you become a better cyclist, it will be the small things that make your cycling more pleasant and rewarding. This chapter will be about some of the techniques that will improve your cycling and your confidence.

Many riders, including some racers, have a devil of a time getting into toe clips. I've seen some straddle the bike, actually placing one foot in the toe clip before they get started. That is one way to do it. You can also simply flip over the pedal cage once the bike starts moving, pedal ten or so revolutions with that foot to give you some speed, and do the same with the other foot. If the second foot is difficult to insert in the toe clip, reach down and do it with your hand, but don't take your eyes off the road. Depending on the circumstances you can tighten the straps or wait. I usually leave them loose until I'm clear of most traffic. It's not uncommon during a group ride for the body to approach a red light and one cyclist will simply topple over because he has forgotten to loosen the straps. The National Team coaches require that team members put one foot on the ground whenever they stop for a light primarily so that riders will get practice putting the foot back in. The truth of the matter is that the team members I have seen can balance their bikes with a rocking movement without getting out of the toe clips, but that is further down the road.

During your training rides there will be times that you must take one or both hands off the handlebars. You might want to reach in your jersey pocket for a banana or zip up your windbreaker. If you must remove one hand for whatever reason, slide the occupied hand over as close as possible to the stem, which will give you better control than if the hand is at the end of the bar. If you hit a bump or pebble in that condition, your bike will likely pull in the direction of the weight.

There is probably no absolutely safe way to ride no hands, but if you want to try it, make sure your frame is not bent or headset pitted, which can be determined by lifting the front wheel off the ground and turning the handlebars. If the steering seems particularly tight in one position, you should have a mechanic check your headset.

The no-hands maneuver should be practiced on a flat, open road with few obstructions and far from fellow cyclists. When you are warmed up and have momentum, remove your hands lightly from the bars. If your frame is not out of alignment you should be able to track in a straight line without consequence. While you should not cycle without hands when you are in the middle of a pack or use the technique capriciously, there is nothing wrong with taking your hands off the bars from time to time, and stretching your back and arms. Consider the technique another part of the arsenal of devices you use to keep your riding time enjoyable.

Group Riding.   In training you will certainly do a great deal of riding on your own, but seize every opportunity to cycle with those who are faster than you. Nothing will improve your speed or improve your technique as quickly. When riding with a handful or a group, you will usually find yourself in a paceline, a move that strings out riders in a straight line with each cyclist taking a turn "pulling" at the front. As with other aspects of cycling, there is an established etiquette of the paceline.

If you've ever had the opportunity to watch the team pursuit, an Olympic event that pits two four-man teams which start on opposite sides of a velodrome, you will likely marvel at how close the pursuiters stay to the wheel in front. Rarely do they move farther back than a few inches. When they have taken their pull—usually half the distance around a 333-meter track—they swing up the banking and slide down behind the third rider. And the beautiful ritual begins all over again.

The kind of pacing most of them do with friends or cycling associates takes place on the roads and is a far more mundane version than the above which the pursuiters have practiced for many thousands of miles. As a training device a paceline is useful because it keeps you going at a pretty good clip and provides little opportunity for loafing. You can, of course, keep company with cyclists who maintain a very fast paceline and whose sole aim is to leave all other riders in their tracks. No sense in keeping company with them.

But if you know the riders and have agreed in advance what pace you will hold and what distance you will travel, then put a paceline on your training schedule. I should add that knowing the other cyclists—meaning you've spent an appreciable amount of time cycling with them and know their habits, quirks and bike-handling ability—is essential. At the time of this writing I am nursing a bad hip bruise because I didn't know another rider's wheel. It is easy to overlap wheels if you are not sure of the movements of the bike in front of you.

The best way to become familiar with pace work is to find a friend you're comfortable with and with whom you have cycled a fair distance. Then find a flat stretch of road where you can move at a brisk pace—15 mph, staying between a foot and six inches from the wheel in front. Until you are comfortable with this close order drill you'll find it a little unsettling. But relax and concentrate.

Owen Mulholland, exracer and cycling journalist, recommends that you develop a split-level vision. "One eye is on the wheel in front and the other is on the road searching for potholes, dogs, intersections, hills and all the myriad elements which can cause the person in front of you to suddenly alter pace. Eventually you can focus almost all attention ahead on the road and practically sense the correct distance behind the front rider."

By all means don't try to be an Olympic team pursuiter during your first paceline ride. Stay a safe distance behind the following wheel until you are sure of yourself and of the person in front. After you've had your turn at the front—and the length you pull and at what speed should have been determined before the ride started—you will normally swing off smoothly to the left, first checking for traffic.

Part of the ride leader's responsibility is to position himself or herself in a slot in relation to the direction of the wind. If the wind is blowing to the right, he should be as far out in the road as safety and prudence permit, allowing the other riders to fan out behind him. If the wind is blowing to the left, the opposite would apply. Clearly this is an ideal circumstance. Traffic and road conditions will likely keep you in a straighter line. Again, don't join a paceline until you are sure of your bike-handling abilities. And always watch out for the other guy. When joining a paceline, announce yourself by saying, "On your wheel," so the rider in front of you knows your intentions.

Hills. There is no easy way over a hill, but certain techniques will make your job a little easier. Technique is often dictated by physiology. Thin riders with favorable

muscle-to-weight ratios can usually climb quickly because
of their high percentage of muscle. These are natural
climbers, like the Colombians who always win the mountains at the Coors Classic Bicycle Race in Colorado. Most
of us have to work at it.

Olympic cyclist Tom Prehn tries to get to the base of
the hill before the climbers so he can catch them on the
way down. Because he is not a natural hill climber, he has
to work on his strategy:

> I tend to use slightly higher gears and lower rpm than
> many of my national teammates. With a lower ca-
> dence a rider needs to sit back more on the saddle,
> concentrating on the power stroke. Upper body strength
> is utilized more with a higher gear (slower rpm). Pull
> back on the bars while pushing forward and down on
> the pedals. The lower back muscles are put to work
> here too. Upper body movement is inevitable and
> even beneficial while climbing hard, as you use your
> weight and upper body strength to propel yourself
> uphill.

The National Team coaches recommend a 60- to 80-rpm
range for climbing hills, a little higher than what Prehn is
suggesting. Over the long run you will conserve energy if
you stay in the saddle during a climb. Your emphasis
should be on spinning and less on the power stroke. But
whatever gear you use, you will likely want to get out of
the saddle from time-to-time if only to relieve your rear
end. Your butt bears the brunt on the hills.

When climbing out of the saddle your hands should
naturally be positioned in the brake levers, cradled in the
slot rather than holding tight. As you push down with
your right leg you pull with the right arm, thus gaining
leverage. Your bike will rock from side to side in a kind of
quiet rhythm. Avoid heavy swaying motions that will sap

your energy and cause you to wander over the face of the road. Research conducted at the University of Manchester, England, has shown that tilting the bike does not seem to offer any great advantage, except for relieving some of the pressure on the arms (*Journal of Biomechanics*, Vol. 12, pp. 527-541, 1979).

You gain some advantages if you climb out of the saddle as a conscious cycling technique rather than as a desperate move to make the crest. Since you are using your legs differently, you are actually stretching and resting them to a degree. And, if it means anything to you, climbing out of the saddle usually enables you to use a bit higher gear, which is probably more important to cyclists who attack hills.

Still, to be able to power up a hill, particularly after a long descent, represents a kind of exhilaration. But I'm talking about late-season exertion, or "honking" here. That is not the kind of thing that you want to do early in the season.

Curt Bond, colleague, cyclist and probably one of the toughest hill climbers in the East, recommends that you train for hills as you would any other terrain. He suggests that you "Do a climb from 200 to 800 feet twice a week. Time each climb and incorporate this into your normal riding. If you don't have any climbs, it may help to train by using big gears into the wind."

He also recommends that

> When sitting, the top half of your body should be relaxed. Concentrate on breathing from your diaphragm and on using a full pedaling motion. Riding with your hands on the drops in an aerodynamic position at these slow speeds is not necessary. Ride on the tops for better breathing.
>
> When standing, your hands should be on the brake

hood for easier breathing. Take a mental check to be sure you are pulling up on the pedals, not just pushing down. Keep your center of gravity over the bottom bracket for more power; resist pushing your body forward over the handlebars. Any violent throwing of the bike from side to side or other exaggerated motion should be avoided for maximum efficiency, especially with a loaded bike. Cycling cleats are a must for any serious climbing.

Riding Light.   Most flat tires—and bent rims—occur in the rear because riders usually place most of their weight over the rear wheels, which can increase when going over obstructions. What you want to do when going over tracks or potholes is get out of the saddle and flex your knees and elbows, centering your weight between the two wheels.

I've always been thrilled by—and sometimes tried to emulate—racers who literally fly over railroad tracks, rather than creep over at odd angles like most humans. The reasons racers can do this is not that they sprout wings; rather, they have learned to lift their bikes by pulling up on the handlebars and pedals, a practice that takes considerable practice.

Olympian Prehn, a very good bike handler, suggests that you

Practice this at a very slow speed until you get the hang of it. A low curb or a speed-trap bump will help you in your timing and coordination. At a walking pace, ride up to the curb. At the instant before the front tire hits it, jerk up sharply on the handlebars. Essentially, you should be lifting the wheel up onto the curb. Do the same thing for the rear wheel: with your crankarms horizontal, jerk up on the pedals the instant before the rear tire catches the curb.

Crossing railroad tracks, the bane of so many cyclists, requires a little more finesse and coordination. Standard advice tells you to cross railroad tracks at a ninety degree angle, which can create some difficulties when the tracks do not form a right angle with the road. In that case you are obliged to form the right angle with your bike and cross the tracks, only after you've checked for traffic.

During a race or training, cyclists often jump a set of tracks, usually after a descent, by pulling up on the bars and pedals simultaneously when the front wheel almost reaches the first track. Timing is crucial, so is velocity. If you're not going at any appreciable speed, you should not try this or when there is a double set of tracks. This is a maneuver for the experts. If in doubt, don't try it.

The point here is that the way you ride and sit on your bike has some bearing on how much road shock your body absorbs and how long your equipment will last. Make a habit of anticipating potholes and minor obstructions. Your legs are better shock absorbers than your butt, so raising yourself off the seat a fraction of an inch when you are passing over some rocky roads will pay dividends in the long run.

I'm really talking about riding "light" rather than "heavy." I'm talking about the little things that will improve the quality of your ride and make the bike more responsive to your handling. To ride light, to ride smart, means being in control of the bike at all times. For example, beginners are notorious for leaning on their brakes. At the start of large recreational rides I've participated in, the only music I've heard for the first couple of miles comes from brake pads rubbing against the rims. On the other hand, even under some of the most treacherous cycling conditions—steep descent and hairpin turns—racers will rarely use their brakes. For a number of years there have been races along the Boardwalk at Atlantic or Ocean City, the course actually being a tight rectangle with the ocean front serving as the homestretch. On these courses there are four ninety-degree turns though you will seldom hear the brakes engaged.

For these cyclists the brakes, which are kept in excellent adjustment, are used sparingly, as a last resort. That is one of the reasons you see many racers cradle the brakes, applying pressure with the index finger, touching them, "feathering" them. Connie Carpenter, an excellent woman racer, has said that one thing she likes about Sue Novara-Reber, ex-World Champion on the track, is that, when there appear to be problems in the riding pack, she motors away from trouble. Very likely the response of the new rider would be to apply the brakes hard in a similar circumstance.

If you are a conscientious cyclist you will read the road and anticipate problems. That habit will reduce your dependence on brakes. Consider that you will likely have much better control of the bike when you are accelerating as compared to when you are braking hard. Touch your brakes, feather them to slow you down. If you are riding in a group, try to use them sparingly. By anticipating your moves and those of others you will use your brakes less.

Stress. During the last seven years I've had the opportunity to attend international cycling events and observe the behavior of cyclists from other nations, particularly Russia and the German Democratic Republic. Much that's derogatory has been written about the super-athletes from these nations; I for one suspect their successes can be attributed more to hard training than to steroids.

At a July 1982 track cycling event I observed the Russian and East Germans prior to their events. To a man (no women in these events) they seemed composed and relaxed. On the other hand, the Americans appeared nervous, skittish, with the exception of a couple of riders who have participated in many international events.

American cyclists are finally learning what their Eastern counterparts have known for years. All things being equal it is often the rider who can control stress who wins the event, particularly in short-distance track events, though antistress techniques have implications for road riders as well. Ed Burke, a Doctor of Physiology and trainer for the American Olympic team, has outlined the methods used at the Training Center.

To reduce tensions he recommends that you begin with a 20-minute period during which you tighten and relax the muscle groups. Lie down in a quiet place and think about relaxation, be conscious of the process. Make fists and be aware of the tension. Do the same thing with your forehead: Tighten and relax. Then with your eyes, face, chest, biceps, thighs, lower legs and feet. Take a deep breath and feel tension leave your body. Burke recommends that cyclists repeat the tensing and relaxing of muscle three times in all.

Building on techniques developed by Dr. Richard Suinn of Colorado State University, Burke recommends that athletes begin an imagery process after the relaxation period. He outlined the procedure in *Velo-News*, a journal of bicycle racing:

1. Remaining quiet, take the first pleasant thought that comes and build upon it. Use it to become more relaxed and dwell upon it for 10 to 15 seconds.

2. Repeat this once or twice.

3. Select an element of the event you are preparing for or wish to practice. It may be the initial burst of the kilometer, the pull at the front during a 100-meter time trial, etc. Remain relaxed.

4. Switch on the scene (for example, just before the start command in the kilometer). Breathe deeply, retain the scene, and continue to let the body relax.

5. Practice in imagery the skill you wish to execute to

precision. Feel the motions as if everything were right on and this were a gold medal race.

6. Make sure to complete the entire skill before you stop. Never practice a mistake.

7. Until your imagery technique develops, use short scenes. Then gradually lengthen them as long as you can remain calm and in charge of the process.

"Through this technique pre-race stress can be reduced and an actual improvement in performance gained. The imagery technique can be used to perform under stress, in poor conditions of environment (bad roads, rain, gusting winds) and during injury rehabilitation."

You might think that, as a casual recreational cyclist, your needs are a far cry from those of America's elite cyclists. While that may be true, you can also learn from their techniques. Whether you are preparing for a century or a long ride, a club race or a personal time trial, you should be as relaxed as possible on the bike. Actually, the relaxation procedure outlined here is pretty standard and is frequently recommended to reduce stress. The imagery process is tied to your performance or the expectations you have for yourself. It stands to reason that you will perform better *in any event* if you are relaxed and have a clear objective. Through imagery you can concentrate on your pedaling or on your breathing, making conscious activities unconscious.

The more you relax on a bike, the better you will feel and perform. You will have moved beyond a literal concern about seat height and stem length to the point that you are thinking about your body moving, getting stronger and overcoming obstacles that might have otherwise curtailed your cycling. Cyclists frequently talk about upgrading their bikes. Well, as you upgrade your bike, be sure to upgrade yourself. As the machine becomes lighter beneath you, in turn you should become lighter on top, perhaps both in composition and attitude. You will most likely lose weight as a consequence of your riding. And you will likely become lighter in spirit as well. The side effects are contagious.

Nick H. Edwards, a dentist from Grand Junction, Tennessee, wrote that during medical school he drove himself hard. At age 26 he developed heart palpitations due to premature ventricular contractions. This led to anxiety and Edwards took tranquilizers and cardiac medications, though he really knew his problems were tied to his personality. He was an overachiever who couldn't relax.

Coaxed by a friend, he purchased a used Schwinn and became hooked on cycling. "The side effects," he writes, "are all constructive—mentally, spiritually, and physically. I have no more palpitations and my EKG is normal; my physician is relieved at my complete recovery. I know my problem has a mixed etiology from the mental and the physical, so when I cycle the words of Maxwell Maltz [author of Psycho-cybernetics] become especially appropriate: 'Happiness is a mental habit, a mental attitude, and if it is not learned and practiced in the present it will never be experienced. It can not be contingent upon solving some external problem.'"

As with Dr. Edwards, countless people have discovered the rhythm of the bicycle, which is more than simply turning the pedals. This rhythm is a fitness born in the body but felt in the mind. And that is total fitness.

12

Measuring Your Health and Fitness

Writing in *Sports Illustrated*, Barry McDermott claims that "Bicycle racers are nuts. They risk their lives and abuse their bodies. On the one hand, they are treated like thoroughbreds: trained, rubbed down and pampered. On the other, they are pushed like tractor trailers: raced day after day until their wheels start smoking."

McDermott was writing about the Coors Classic, the finest stage-race in America, though he could be talking about any race, anytime. Are racers nuts? Perhaps, but certainly they are some of the fittest nuts around. And the distance between the fast recreational cyclist and the racer is more than just 10 miles an hour; it's a quality of dedication and commitment to the sport far beyond any winner's purse. You might never choose to be a racer—yet you can certainly learn something from racers about fitness. If you want to go beyond the kind of fitness I've been writing about so far, listen to the experts.

How do you know you're fit? Good question. Obvious measures of fitness include reduced resting and increased training pulse, greater oxygen uptake and generally improved circulation. You will know the anecdotal signs; hills will be easier to climb, you will be able to ride distances at a high cadence without feeling fatigued.

If you have been cycling for at least a season and are

putting in a couple of hundred miles a week with specialty training, such as intervals, can you qualify your fitness? Is there a way to put a numerical value on your level of fitness—aside from the casual glance at the bathroom scale?

As I've said throughout this book, taking your pulse is one of the best ongoing measurements of your fitness. Weight loss (or reduction in body fat) is another, and comparing your cholesterol level now to when you started four or five months ago will tell you a lot.

But now let's go a bit further.

TRACKING YOUR FITNESS

Coach Norman Sheil is a great believer in keeping a diary and he has given that advice to many of the champions he has coached. He strongly recommends his racers record their weight and sleep habits each day. As well as recording the pulse rate on waking, Sheil places emphasis on the pulse-recovery rate and suggests using the Harvard Step Test, a simple and reliable indicator, to determine your fitness level.

The Harvard Step Test. To perform the step test you will need a 20-inch-high bench. Step up and down thirty times a minute to a count of four: first foot up, second foot up; first foot down; second foot down. Continue the exercise for five minutes, or less if exhaustion sets in. Then sit down and take your pulse at the following intervals: 1–1½ minutes, 2–2½ minutes, 3–3½ minutes. Determine your Physical Efficiency Index based on this formula:

$$\frac{\text{Duration of Exercise in Seconds} \times 100}{2 \times \text{Sum of Three Pulse Counts}} = \text{Physical Efficiency}$$

An example:

$$\frac{300 \times 100}{2 \times (75 + 50 + 35)} = 94$$

For the training cyclists coach Shiel provides the following ranges and ratings.

Above 90—Excellent
From 80–89—Good
From 65–79—High Average
From 55–64—Low Average
Below 55—Poor

Keeping in mind that pulse rate varies significantly with age and level of training, you should not compare yourself to the above figures. For example, if you are a 30-year-old male, you are not likely to have the same recovery pulse reading of a younger man. If you had pulse readings of 80, 60 and 50, you'd have a score of 78, which would be very good for you.

As Sheil points out, the value of the test is not to attain a high score but for you to measure improvement as your training progresses. *Don't put yourself in competition with bicycle racers: Compete against yourself.* The better your training, the quicker you will recover from exercise. That is a very personal thing. The only competition is yourself.

The Harvard Step Test is a fairly simple way to measure your cardiovascular fitness, an important yardstick. If you would like a more sophisticated system, consider that used by the U.S. National Team. Again, I offer this as an example and a guide; not an absolute you should measure your performance against. And this fitness test is certainly not for you if you have not already achieved a high level of fitness and completed the program already outlined in this book.

Progressive Resistance Test.   For years the U.S. National Team has been trying to quantify exactly how fit our best cyclists are. For most of us, we can pay attention to how many miles we ride in an hour or how fast we ride a century and get a reasonably good measure of our fitness. I have a 38-mile ride that I complete in about 2 hours and 20 to 27 minutes usually, a reasonably good measure of our capabilities. But our elite cyclists needed a better yardstick. To that end National Coach Eddy Borysewicz and Sports Medicine Director Ed Burke devised a progressive resistance test to be conducted on the Monarch ergometer, a stationary bicycle. While a very useful test for competitive cyclists, it was not generally applicable because a lot of people didn't have access to an ergometer, except through a YMCA or health club. (If you have access to an ergometer, I encourage you to use it.)

To make this test applicable to the club rider and all those interested in fitness, Ken Myer and David F. Fayran devised a similar system but one to be used on a Racer Mate, an indoor exercise device that is readily available; you can also use another popular product, the Turbo Trainer. Both are available at your local bike shop. This fitness test can be taken in your home with some assistance. Also, cycling clubs frequently purchase a Racer Mate (price: $45) for the club's use. You must use it on the stand that comes with the Racer Mate.

PHASE 1
Before you begin your fitness evaluation you should have some help to assist you in taking measurements. Take your resting heart rate and blood pressure and record them in accompanying chart. I'm assuming that by this time, if

you are interested in your total fitness you will have access to a sphygmomanometer for blood pressure readings. I personally think one belongs in every medicine kit. And it's no more complicated than taking your pulse.

Next you should warm up, spinning at about 90 rpm in a 70-inch gear for six minutes. After six minutes your associate should record your heart rate while you are pedaling. You will also record your Total Work Units (TWU) based on the following conversion. Note that the figure for TWUs has already been calculated.

PHASE 2
In this phase you should spin the pedals at 90 rpm in an 82-inch gear (52 x 17) for the next five minutes, until you're eleven minutes into the test. For this you earn 1,505 Total Work points a minute for a total of 7,525. Have your associate record your heart rate eleven minutes into the test while you continue to pedal.

PHASE 3
Increase the cadence to 100 rpm in a 90-inch gear (50 x 15) for five minutes until you reach the sixteen-minute mark. Record your heart rate. Add 11,410 Total Work Units.

PHASE 4
Increase your gear to 94 inches (52 x 15) at 100 rpm and continue to exhaustion. You will earn 2,734 Total Work Units per minute (or fraction of a minute). Record finishing time and heart rate. Then record heart rate at one, two, and three minute intervals after you finish, even if you have not fully completed the first three stages.

Add the heart rates from one, two and three minutes. And use the following formula:

$$\frac{\text{Total Work (TW)} \times \text{Percentage of Work Completed}}{\text{Total Heart Rate } (1 + 2 + 3)}$$

Your percentage of work completed should be based on sixteen minutes. Fourteen minutes would be 87.5% and so on.

Example:

If you ride sixteen minutes you will earn 24,401 TWU. If, for example, your recorded heart rates for the three minutes are 139, 90 and 75 beats totaling 304, your total would be:

$$\frac{24,401 \text{ TW} \times 100\%}{304 \text{ heartbeats}} = 8,026 \text{ points}$$

You might not complete the sixteen-minute test program. If you don't, divide the amount of time completed by sixteen minutes. For example, if your points total 17,555 and you cycled thirteen minutes (81% of 16):

$$\frac{17,555 \times 81\%}{304 \text{ heartbeats}} = 4,677 \text{ points}$$

TABLE EIGHT

TURBO TRAINER CONVERSION

1st Step	$78'' = 52 \times 18$
2nd Step	$90'' = 50 \times 15$
3rd Step	$100'' = 52 \times 14$
4th Step	$103'' = 53 \times 14$

TABLE NINE

CONVERSIONS

Minutes	Load	Cadence	Total Work/Minute (Kilogram-meters/min.)
0 - 6	70" (52 × 20)	90 rpm	911 (× 6 = 5,466)
6 - 11	82" (52 × 17)	90 rpm	1505 (× 5 = 7,525)
11 - 16	90" (50 × 15)	100 rpm	2282 (× 5 = 11,410)
16-exhaustion	94" (52 × 15)	100 rpm	2734

Sum of Total Work Units at 16 minutes = 24,401 = 100% of work completed.

TABLE TEN

TEST RESULTS

Test Date	Weight	Resting		70" 90 rpm 1-6 min.	82" 90 rpm 6-11 min.	90" 100 rpm 11-16 min.
		Heart Rate	Blood Pressure	H.R.	H.R.	H.R.

After you have determined your point total, what do the numbers mean? Here are the scores for classes of National Team riders.

 5,000 points = Excellent for junior men (under 18 years)
 8,000 points = Good for senior men (over 18 years)
10,000 points = Excellent for senior men
 3,000 points = Good for women
 5,000 points = Excellent for women

These points are for national caliber riders so be careful of comparisons. Some racers scored as low as 4,876 points for 16 minutes and as high as 15,092 for 22 minutes.

What you earn in the way of points will depend on the level of fitness you bring to this test. Obviously, this isn't a test to be taken casually by a recreational cyclist; it was designed for national team cyclists and should only be undertaken if you already have a high level of fitness—and if you have some help. You might want to join a club which has use of a Racer Mate or to take this test at your local YMCA or health club. It is important that your performance is monitored. If you have a Turbo Trainer, use the accompanying conversion table to figure out your gearing for the various phases.

No matter what the point total is, keep in mind that your only competition is yourself—*not the national team*. Take the test a few times, particularly after you have a solid background of mileage and specialty training, perhaps at the end of the season. Then you might want to try again early the next year, particularly if you have maintained your level of fitness with winter training, the subject of a later chapter.

The VO$_2$ Test. A determination of your total fitness would probably require facilities not generally available to everyone. By knowing your pulse, your recovery rate, and your lean-to-fat body ratio you will have a good idea of your level of fitness. Another important measure is VO$_2$ testing to determine maximum oxygen consumption, though you usually can't get this kind of service at your local YMCA.

Physiologists consider that the VO$_2$ test is one of the best indicators of an endurance athlete's level of fitness and potential because it tells you how much oxygen is actually being taken up by the muscles. The accompanying chart gives mean scores for elite cyclists (oxygen consumption as expressed in milliliters of oxygen per kilogram of body weight per minute).

TABLE ELEVEN

VO$_2$ SCORES OF ELITE CYCLISTS

Study	Number of Subjects	VO$_2$ Max (ml^2/kg/min)
U.S. Men's National Team	23	74.0
Norwegian National Team	16	73.0
Swedish National Team, 1975	5	69.1
National Class Road and Track Cyclists	11	67.1
U.S. Women's National Team	6	57.4
U.S. Category One Men	8	70.6
U.S. Junior National Team	15	64.8

Courtesy of Ed Burke

Again, don't compare yourself with National Team members. You should know that as your weight and body fat decrease, your VO$_2$ uptake will probably increase too, which will make a demonstrable difference in your training and hill climbing. *Bicycling* magazine commissioned Ed Pavelka, cyclist and sports journalist, to have a VO$_2$ test at an area hospital. Pavelka, who is 36 and six-four, weighed 84 kilograms when he was first tested and had a VO$_2$ maximum of 52. During the next four weeks he rode 950 miles, reduced his weight to 80.5 kilograms and his body fat to 11 percent. At this time his VO$_2$ reading was 59. Even had his aerobic level remained constant, the weight loss would have improved his oxygen uptake.

If you are a serious cyclist and want to know more about yourself than pulse, blood pressure and weight readings offer, you can get a full-fledged exam performed in a sport medicine facility at your local hospital or university. For about $120 you can get a VO$_2$ max text, a lung capacity measurement, and a body fat measurement. As fitness and fitness measurement become more institutionalized, these services will likely be more available.

Electronic Fitness Monitoring. To keep track of your training on a day-to-day basis, you might consider purchase of an electronic monitor which can be a very useful training tool while you are cycling.

Bicycling has not escaped the electronic revolution. In the last few years manufacturers have made available a wide range of cadence and heart pulse monitors to help cyclists better monitor their training and performance while riding both indoors and out. Because the technology is changing so rapidly, I will point out some generic features and a few brands.

Some monitors pick up the heart's electrical impulse through electrodes. Others record the flow of blood through the vessels with infrared light. Both heart and pulse monitors can be equally reliable, though individual brands differ markedly depending on circuitry and design. If you intend to use your monitor strapped to the handlebars while you are cycling outside, you will want one that can withstand the rain and the road. You'll also want a unit that is fairly light.

Some of these units, such as the Genesis Exercise Computer, are worn like a wristwatch with a calculator to program your pre-exercise pulse and an alarm to tell you if you are working too hard or easily. It also provides a metronome to help you set cadence. Your pulse is taken by a small sensor strapped to your left index finger.

Other units, such as the Amerec Pulse Meter, are secured to the handlebars. A wire runs from the computer to your earlobe to pick up the pulse. With most units mounted on the bars you simply slip a finger into a sensor and take a pulse reading.

There are a number of heart monitors available. Units that are strapped to your chest and through electrodes monitor your heartbeat. Although these can be used when cycling outside, cyclists seem to prefer these for indoor use.

With such a selection of units on the market, which one should you buy, if any? Price is obviously a consideration. At this writing pulse monitors cost from $50 to $100 depending on the features. But prices are falling.

Ease of use and versatility are other considerations. Does the unit mount securely on your handlebars and can you read your pulse without difficulty while you are riding?

How much data you want to deal with is yet another consideration. Some of these units can be preprogrammed to signal you at various pulse rate levels, depending on the kind of workout you want. You might find that these electronic gizmos clutter up your bike and cycling experience, and you'd rather rely on traditional pulse-taking measures.

On the other hand, these units—usually weighing less than a pound—will make you much more conscious of your cycling. You will have a visible reminder of when you are loafing; you will also have a handy guide to assist you with interval training. Ultimately, it depends on what kind of cycling you intend to do. If you want to get the fullest possible benefit from your cycling, if you intend to go on a vigorous fitness program complete with daily diary entries, a pulse or heart monitor would be in order.

Before you put your money down, a word about reliability. You will gain no benefit if the unit is not accurately recording your pulse. To determine the reliability of a cross-section of models, *Bicycling* magazine tested the readings from these monitors against readings obtained from an electrocardiogram (EKG) with the help of a cardiopulmonary technician at a local hospital. By and large we found the monitors fairly accurate ranging from ± 1.3% to ± 9.1%.

A word of caution. That figure can be misleading. If you use the monitor incorrectly—for instance, if you move your hand while taking a reading—you could get a very significant fluctuation.

Measuring your level of fitness should not be a comparative analysis. What someone else does on a test should be of little consequence to you. The important thing is your progress. You will recall in some of the earlier success stories individuals who could hardly walk were able to pedal a bike around the block, then around town. In time, they were doing centuries. What better indication of fitness and progress can one ask for?

On the other hand, as your level of fitness increases, your improvement, while real, is likely to be incremental. For that reason it is important to have a specific riding and training schedule and to somehow monitor your performance. The easiest way to do this is with a diary, where you would note daily mileage, pulse, weight, and eating habits, a practice that takes minutes. Depending on your inclination and your willingness to play with gadgets, an electronic pulse monitor might be just the thing to help you maintain cadence and reach your training pulse rate.

There are other electronic gadgets designed to measure your fitness and performance. Specifically, these are devices usually weighing less than half a pound that you attach to your handlebars. These lightweight computers can be purchased at most bike shops for anywhere from $40 to $70. Some popular models are the Pacer 2000, Entex Bike Computer, the Cyclocomputer, the Digi-Speed, the Avocet Cyclometer, the Veltec, Peugot's Sport Computer, Cyclotron, Push, Coach and many more.

Electronic aids offer a range of benefits and services, including: speed, distance, total mileage, average speed, maximum speed, cadence and more. For example, you can inform the Bike Computer how far you plan to ride and how long you'd like to take and ask it to calculate the speed you'll have to maintain. You can even get optional heart rate and cadence monitors. The Coach measures oxygen uptake and calorie expenditure.

Again, these computers won't do the work for you, though they will make you more conscious of your cadence, speed, and total mileage. As in fishing, it is not uncommon for a cyclist to overstate his or her mileage or miles per hour. A computer can help keep us honest.

How elaborate a system you purchase will depend on your needs and preferences. I find it very helpful to have a readout of my cadence and mph, especially when I'm on a designated training ride. If I'm out for a leisurely spin with my family, those matters are far less important.

Keep in mind that this field is changing very quickly, for the good, I think. Since the first units were introduced five years ago, manufacturers have significantly improved the products, making them very useful for cyclists interested in monitoring their fitness while on a bike.

13

Food for Fitness

I've just heard a television announcer say that Tour de France riders consume more than 9,000 calories a day during that grueling 20-plus-day event of more than 2,000 miles.

With that kind of energy requirement, you'd think it wouldn't matter what kind of foods the Tour riders consume—but it does. As American professional Greg LeMond points out, the riders stay away from a lot of greasy food and red meat because these choices will likely hurt their performance.

America has known for at least a decade that "you are what you eat." Or, as they say in the computer business, "Garbage in, garbage out." What you eat will affect your performance on a bike, whether you are taking a long tour or riding a century. Furthermore, if exercise is a lifetime habit with a lifetime of reward, you should put the same value on diet. We all know plenty of cyclists (or runners or softball players) who seem to defy the laws of energy metabolism; they eat and drink a lot of beer but never get fat. I think part of the reason for this is that many are in their 20s and 30s and maintaining an ambitious exercise schedule. You can burn off a lot of calories if you're getting seven to eight hours of strenuous exercise each week.

But the beauty of exercise, as I have indicated, is that

you can earn some fairly substantial rewards with little investment of time. However, if you plan to cycle three hours a week, all the more reason to watch what you eat. If you operate on the assumption that exercise is a license to eat anything you want, then you'd better plan to spend a lot of time on your bike.

Bob Howells of Indiana, who had more than twenty years' cycling experience and had volunteered to lead a group on a 100-mile ride, learned the hard way about good nutrition one day when his group had to turn back at the halfway point because many of the beginners showed up without food or water.

"Some cyclists thought they'd lose weight on the trip so they skipped breakfast altogether. Others ate something beforehand and figured they'd need no food or water during the ride. They just didn't realize how important food is while cycling. You need to eat well before going out on any long rides and it's essential to take along plenty of snacks to give you energy," Howells said.

He tried sharing his granola bars, sandwiches and fruit with the group but they weren't enough. And the evidence was in the pace, which got slower and slower after twenty miles. No gear was low enough.

Howells' experience convinced his local cycling club to make a firm rule: No cyclists can participate without an adequate supply of food and water. While this is a sensible rule for you to follow, good nutrition really begins long before you get on your bike. The right diet will improve your cycling performance and give you the energy to work toward your goals.

As with weight loss, I'm not going to engage in magic here. Your best way to get a balanced diet is by eating several servings from the four basic food groups, including two or more servings of meat or other protein sources;

four or more of bread, pastas, and grains; four or more of fruits and vegetables; and two or more of milk and other dairy products (see Table Twelve).

In an earlier chapter I suggested you keep a diary to record your mileage, pulse and other vital factors. If you are particularly interested in weight loss and significant performance on a bike, you might also keep a record of what you eat, at least for a few weeks, longer if you really want to understand how your body works.

All cyclists from beginner to professional should eat plenty of carbohydrates—up to 60–65 percent of your total diet. Both complex carbohydrates (starches), found in whole-grain bread and pastas, and simple carbohydrates (sugars), found in fruits and candy, are broken down in the body and used by the muscles for energy. You should eat the whole grains and dried legumes (lentils, kidney beans, and peas) which are good sources of carbohydrates and of B vitamins that help metabolize the carbohydrates for energy. There's no need for the fitness cyclists to avoid cakes and cookies, though they do lack the other nutrients that complex carbohydrates provide. Know yourself and know what you're eating.

TABLE TWELVE

THE BASIC FOUR—A NEW AMERICAN EATING GUIDE

GROUP	ANYTIME	IN MODERATION	NOW AND THEN
1 BEANS GRAINS NUTS *Four or more servings a day*	bread and rolls (whole grain) bulgar dried beans and peas (legumes) lentils oatmeal whole wheat pasta brown rice rye bread sprouts whole grain hot and cold cereals whole wheat matzoh	cornbread granola cereals hominy grits macaroni and cheese matzoh nuts pasta, except whole wheat peanut butter pizza unsweetened cereals refried beans, commercial or home-made in oil seeds soybeans waffles or pancakes with syrup white bread and rolls white rice	croissant doughnut (yeast-leavened) presweetened breakfast cereals sticky buns stuffing (made with butter)

GROUP	ANYTIME	IN MODERATION	NOW AND THEN
GROUP 2 FRUITS VEGE-TABLES *Four or more servings a day*	all fruits and vegetables, except those listed at right applesauce (unsweetened) unsweetened fruit juices unsalted vegetable juices white or sweet potatoes	avocado coleslaw cranberry sauce dried fruit french fries, homemade in vegetable oil or commercial fried eggplant (in vegetable oil) fruits canned in syrup gazpacho glazed carrots guacamole potatoes au gratin salted vegetable juices sweetened fruit juices vegetables canned with salt	coconut pickles

GROUP	ANYTIME	IN MODERATION	NOW AND THEN
GROUP 3 MILK PRODUCTS *Adults:* *2 servings a day* *Children:* *3 to 4 servings a day*	buttermilk made from low-fat cottage cheese low-fat milk, 1% milkfat low-fat yogurt nonfat dry milk skim milk cheeses skim milk skim milk and banana shake	cocoa made with skim milk cottage cheese, regular, 4% milkfat frozen low-fat yogurt ice milk low-fat milk, 2% milkfat low-fat yogurt, sweetened mozzarella cheese, part-skim type only	cheesecake cheese fondue cheese soufflé custard eggnog ice cream whipped cream
GROUP 4 POULTRY FISH MEAT EGGS *Two servings a day* [*Vegetarians:* *Nutrients in these*	Fish cod flounder haddock halibut perch pollock rockfish shellfish, except shrimp sole tuna, water-packed Egg Products,	Fish (drained well, if canned) fried fish salmon, pink, canned sardines, shrimp, tuna, oil-packed Poultry chicken liver fried chicken, homemade in vegetable oil	Poultry fried chicken, commercially prepared Egg cheese omelet egg yolk or whole egg (about 3 a week) Red Meats bacon beef liver,

GROUP	ANYTIME	IN MODERATION	NOW AND THEN
foods can be obtained by eating more foods in Groups 1, 2 and 3]	egg whites only Poultry chicken or turkey, boiled, baked or roasted (no skin)	chicken or turkey, boiled, baked or roasted (with skin) Red Meats (trimmed of fat) leg or loin of lamb pork shoulder of loin, lean ground round rump roast beef steak, lean veal	fried bologna corned beef ham, trimmed well hot dogs liverwurst pig's feet salami sausage spareribs untrimmed red meats

Reprinted with permission from the *New American Eating Guide* which is available from Center for Science in the Public Interest, 1755 S St., NW, Washington, D.C. 20009, for $3 ($6 laminated), copyright © 1979.

TABLE THIRTEEN

HIGH-CARBOHYDRATE FOODS FOR THE CYCLE TOURIST

FOOD	CALORIES	CARBOHYDRATES (grams)	FATS (grams)
Apple (1, 3¼" diameter)	123	30.7	1.3
Apple Juice (1 cup)	117	29.5	trace
Banana (1 medium)	101	26.4	0.2
Beans, canned (1 cup)	306	58.7	1.3
Beans, Lima, cooked (1 cup)	189	33.7	0.9
Biscuit (1)	91	14.6	2.6
Bran Muffin (1)	104	17.2	3.9
Bread, whole wheat (1 slice)	61	11.9	0.8
Bulgar, cooked (1 cup)	22.7	47.3	0.9
Cornflakes (1 cup)	97	21.3	0.1
Macaroni, cooked (1 cup)	192	39.1	0.7
Oatmeal, cooked (1 cup)	132	23.3	2.4
Oatmeal, raw (1 cup)	312	54.6	5.9
Orange Juice (1 cup)	112	25.8	0.5
Pancakes (1, 6" diameter)	164	23.7	5.3
Peaches, canned, water-packed (1 cup)	76	19.8	0.2
Pizza, slice (5½" arc)	153	18.4	0.54
Potatoes, boiled and diced (1 cup)	118	26.5	0.2
Potatoes, fried (1 cup)	456	55.4	24.1
Raisins (½ cup)	209	56.1	0.15
Rice, brown, cooked (1 cup)	232	49.7	1.2
Strawberries, raw (1 cup)	55	12.5	0.7
Spaghetti with Tomato Sauce and Cheese (1 cup)	260	37	8.8
Syrup (1 oz.)	99	25.5	—
Wheat Germ, Toasted (1 tbsp)	23	3	0.7

Without any of your gastronomical delights, try to think of the food you eat as fuel, because that's what it is and that's how your body responds. When you are cycling very hard—anaerobically (without oxygen)—such as during a tough hill climb, carbohydrates provide a readily available energy source. In more moderate exercise (aerobic) the body burns both carbohydrates and fats in the presence of oxygen. Thus, on long steady rides, you are burning a mixture of fuels. As you improve your cycling, you will want to take long steady rides to teach your body how to burn fat efficiently at a moderate pace.

But you don't have to eat fat to burn it—don't laugh, I've heard more than one person make that claim. Although the body burns fat for energy, you definitely don't have to emphasize high-fat foods in your diet. Quite the contrary. At best, fats should constitute no more than 25 percent of your total calories. The body can store an awful lot of fat in the adipose and muscle tissue—70,000 calories worth of fat.

On the other hand, the muscles can store about 1,600 calories of carbohydrates in its metabolized form. Simple mathematics will tell you that you must constantly replenish your carbohydrate supply during rides over two hours, the point at which most nutritionists indicate your carbohydrate stores are depleted.

Again, why wait for that big Sunday ride to have a carbohydrate feast: Increase your carbohydrate stores by eating a balanced diet. We know from laboratory tests that cyclists who eat high-carbohydrate diets (55 to 65 percent) perform better and feel less fatigued after cycling. That should be worth something to you.

In one study, athletes maintained a steady pace on a stationary bicycle for 60 minutes following a high fat and protein diet over a two-week period; 115 minutes after a mixed diet which included carbohydrates; and 170 minutes at a steady pace following a high-carbohydrate (at least 65 percent) diet.

At the Grand Forks Human Nutrition Research Center, researchers subjected cyclists to three different diets for three months beginning with a four-week-long diet high (50 percent) in saturated fat; switching to a high (55 percent) carbohydrate menu; and then in the last month eating foods rich (50 percent) in polyunsaturated fat.

Diet significantly influenced performance. The high-carbohydrate menu got the most votes. Volunteers reported feeling and riding better after eating carbohydrate-rich foods such as fruits, vegetables, grains and pastas. Moreover, their vital signs (heart rate and oxygen consumption) returned to normal after strenuous activity more quickly when eating a high-carbohydrate diet. Researcher Hank Lukaski called a high-carbohydrate diet, one which stressed grains and pastas, fruits and vegetables, "ideal" for cyclists. Good food means good health.

The results from the high-fat diet were less impressive. As noted earlier, although our bodies draw on fats as a major fuel source during light to moderate workloads, we certainly don't need to supplement our fat supplies with special diet. In fact, cyclist Steve Tilford reported that while on the high-fat diet at Grand Forks, "I couldn't ride very well eating those high-fat foods like meat, oil and butter. I felt sick most of the time."

In fact, while cycling, there's no point in eating fatty foods like meat or dairy products, as they're apt to sit in the gut for hours. Fats actually stimulate the release of enterogastrone, a hormone which slows digestion. Not surprisingly, racers indicate they purposely avoid fatty or greasy foods. Good food makes good sense.

But that doesn't mean avoid fatty foods altogether. "Don't be afraid of getting a little fat in your diet," advises Tom Dickson, M.D., Medical Director for the Lehigh

County Velodrome in Trexlertown, Pennsylvania. "Most of us eat too much fat, but many cyclists I've seen try to stay away from fat entirely, which is just not good. They don't realize that it contributes significantly to performance, especially during long rides. I'd say a diet of 60 percent carbohydrates, 30 percent fats and 10 percent protein strikes a perfect balance."

By the way, don't make the mistake of thinking that because you're now cycling—and burning up extra calories— that gives you free rein to eat all the high-calorie carbohydrate sweets you like. Excess carbohydrate calories that are not burned off are stored as fat in the adipose tissue. A rapid weight gain is just as tough on cyclists as on anyone else.

Moderation in everything, including carbohydrates and fats, seems to be the key. To help you with your own nutrition program, we've devised a sample menu which emphasizes carbohydrates, fats and proteins in proper proportion. Consider it suggestive rather than definitive. As you become more adept in cycling, and log longer miles, you may want to keep a food diary to keep track of all those meals and snacks shoveled down in an average day. Write down *everything* you eat and how you felt while riding. "And after a few months, you'll be able to see how foods affect your cycling," points out Roy Knickman, a well-known racer who's kept a food diary for years, "and what foods leave you feeling sluggish. I guarantee that if you keep a food diary for six months you'll improve your diet and your riding." And you'll probably lose weight.

The Protein Connection. This emphasis on carbohydrates as an all-important diet and fuel source may come as a surprise to a generation weaned on steaks and prime cuts of beef. But the truth is that a high-protein diet does little to contribute to muscle energy, despite what you may read in the popular press.

In fact, only 10 to 15 percent of our normal daily diet should be comprised of protein; any more, and you'll have problems with performance. The waste products of protein are processed through the kidneys and that extra digestive stress during an activity like cycling can be a hindrance.

Protein *is* important for overall health, however. In fact, human beings are 20 percent protein by weight. The substance makes up our muscles, skin, hair, nails, eyes and teeth, and contributes to the formation of the blood, heart, lungs, brain and nerves. We need a continuous supply of protein to maintain proper cell structure. Hemoglobin, the substance in the blood that transports oxygen from the lungs to the tissues and brings back carbon dioxide to the lungs to be eliminated from the body, is comprised almost totally of protein. More importantly, protein is responsible for the production of enzymes (which aid in the digestion of food) and hormones (which regulate our bodies' processes). Without an ample supply of protein, our bodies wouldn't maintain an adequate balance of fluid.

Besides, while a cyclist may not derive any energy boost from eating yogurt, fish, or other protein sources, proteins make up the composition of our muscles. Every muscle contains filamentous cells, or fibers. Inside the cell membrane are long, parallel rows of contractile proteins, called actin and myosin. These contractile proteins are the smallest moving parts of every cell. Although protein isn't a forerunner in athletes' diets, it does form the base for all muscular development. So be sure to include some protein-rich foods in your diet—meat, eggs, fish, cheese, liver and the like—just don't go overboard.

Just how much protein the cyclist requires on a daily basis is still a matter of debate. Depending on the physician or nutritionist you consult, your suggested daily allowance of protein can range anywhere from one gram per kilogram of body weight (2.2 pounds) to .8 grams per kilogram. For instance, the Food and Nutrition Board of the National Research Council advises individuals to consume at least one gram of protein per kilogram daily, which for a 160-pound athlete totals about 73 grams. On the other hand, some physicians and nutritionists have concluded that .8 grams per kilogram is sufficient.

How does this translate to the food you eat? A six-ounce rib-eye steak, for example, contains 42 grams of protein (one ounce of meat equals seven grams of protein). According to the one gram/kilogram formula, that's not enough for one day, but you can complement your diet by adding other animal or vegetable proteins too.

You may feel confused about these discrepancies in the protein allowances recommended, or may already have found that this one gram/kilogram formula isn't suited to your dietary needs. As you grow more conscious of diet and what foods contribute to your best performance, you become better able to gauge your own protein intake. "You have to know your own body," points out Dale Stetina, a winner of the 1982 Coors Classic. "Some people have a meat-eating metabolism and some don't." He doesn't and it hasn't slowed him down.

In time, you'll probably want to tackle a special event—a race, a century or a multi-day tour. Diet is particularly important in this context.

The week before you ride increase your carbohydrate intake to 60 to 65 percent of your daily diet to elevate the amount of glycogen in the muscle cells.

A high-carbohydrate breakfast such as pancakes and juice works wonders on the morning of a long ride. (Some cyclists like to eat pasta for breakfast before hitting the road; to each his own!) Carbohydrates can be digested and stored within the muscle cells in about two to three hours.

But in long events, particularly those that are longer than two hours, high-carbohydrate snacks are especially important. Research has shown that most carbohydrates (except some high-fiber foods) can start to be transformed into glucose within 50 to 70 minutes of entering the digestive system. While it takes longer to store the glycogen as muscle fuel, it is important to replenish your blood sugar (glucose) supply constantly.

"How quickly you digest food depends on how hard you're working and how full your stomach is, but we do know carbohydrates are digested faster than fats or proteins," points out Ed Burke, national team trainer. "You should replenish your glucose levels with foods easily digested such as fruits, apples, bananas, raisins, dates, small tarts. The important thing is don't wait fifty miles into the ride before you start to drink and eat. Start drinking fluids right away and eat within the first half hour."

TABLE FOURTEEN
SAMPLE MENU FOR CYCLISTS IN TRAINING

Sample Menu	Breakfast	Noon Meal	Evening Meal
Day 1	cereal (1 cup) milk 2% fat (1 cup) toast (3 slices) butter (1 tablespoon) juice (½ cup) beverage	macaroni salad (1 cup) contains macaroni, ½ egg, 2 tablespoons kidney beans, salad oil vegetable (½ cup) bread (3 slices) butter milk, 2% fat (½ cup)	lean meat, poultry or fish (6–8 ounces) potato (½ cup) other vegetable or salad (½ cup) rolls (3) butter cake beverage

Sample Menu	Breakfast	Noon Meal	Evening Meal
Day 2	fresh orange juice (½ cup) whole grain cereal (1 cup) low-fat milk (1 cup) hot zucchini whole wheat muffins (2) butter hot spearmint tea	large salad bowl with dressing contains chick peas, greens, ½ egg, cheese cubes, broccoli, pepper, sprouts bran muffins hot beverage	chicken cacciatore (6–8 ounces) three grain pilaf with mushrooms (½ cup) chilled green beans vinaigrette (½ cup) white wheat rolls (2) butter fresh fruit cup (½ cup) beverage
Day 3	fresh sliced peach oatmeal granola (1 cup) plain yogurt (1 cup) whole wheat pumpkin bread (2 slices) hot orange spice tea	chili (1 cup) contains ground beef, kidney beans, tomato sauce brown rice (1 cup) corn bread (2 slices) fresh pineapple slices cold spring water	broiled bluefish (4 ounces) baked potato with plain yogurt tossed green salad (½ cup) pumpernickel rolls (2) butter apple raisin pie with whole wheat crust hot beverage

Nutritionist Ann Grandjean, who works with the U.S. Olympic Cycling Team, also cautioned against eating foods that are highly sugared while cycling. "Raisins are good, but peanut butter sandwiches are better," she suggests. "Banana-nut bread provides energy, as do tortillas. Cold pasta is nice for a change. Cookies are all right, providing they contain more flour than sugar."

Glucose and the Bonk.

Sometimes the excitement of a ride causes a rider to neglect a high-carbohydrate diet on the road. He or she might roar out of the starting blocks the first day and fall asleep early that evening. The next day, hungry and without momentum, the rider crawls along. Why? Because he has burned up all his glycogen stores and must work to replenish them—which he does by riding cautiously, stopping frequently, and consuming a lot of carbohydrates. Things will get better quickly.

In its extreme form the above incident might affectionately be called "The Bonk," one form of hypoglycemia (low blood sugar). It happened to me once and seemed far worse than "hitting the wall" in a marathon, though I realize both are cousins in fatigue.

I was cycling with a friend from Allentown, Pennsylvania, to Dayton, Ohio. Knowing the rugged Pennsylvania hills awaited us, we decided to push the pace early and get that part of the trip behind us. At about the 110-mile mark, I was climbing yet another hill and found myself completely without energy. I simply stopped pedaling and couldn't go any farther. On reflection I realized that, while we had eaten, we had probably not eaten enough for that amount of cycling. Luckily we found a motel down the road and after a couple of beers I was feeling great again. I ate a lot of carbohydrates that night.

I could have avoided that condition by eating and drinking a little more during the day and resting more often. The exhilaration of cycling can be overwhelming. Don't let it take you for a ride.

Here is Olympic racer Brent Emery's diet plan and some of his favorite recipes:

Daily Diet. "With regular riding, I burn about 3,000 to 4,000 calories a day. The mainstay of my diet is carbohydrates. They're easy to digest and give me energy. But I always eat a good number of foods from all the food groups. I gave up vitamins completely in the 1982 season and didn't seem to suffer for it, but after I got injured I started taking three different kinds of vitamin and mineral supplements every day."

Spring Training. "My year-round diet stresses carbohydrates, but they're especially important in the spring. I eat a lot of complex (slow-burning) carbohydrates, such as brown-rice and pasta for longer-lasting energy. In the summer, I eat more simple carbohydrates (sugars), the kind you find in baked goods, for quicker energy. But I don't go overboard."

Sprints. "I don't like to eat a lot of fat on the day of a sprint because it takes too long to digest. On the morning of a race, I get up early and eat raisins and rice [see recipe]. I won't eat anything two hours before I race because I'm a little more aggressive on an empty stomach. Sheila Young-Ochowicz always races a little hungry and it works well for her."

Stage Races. "I need to eat some meat, chicken, rice, all kinds of solid food before a stage race. [A stage race is a point-to-point race with rests in between.—Au.] These races can really drain your body so you need a good base of nutrition. In the weeks before, I'll ride about 75 to 100 miles a day, get plenty of sleep and massages, and eat from the Basic Four. During the race itself I'll eat some rice cakes and dried fruit. I also like to eat almond bars, a small piece of candy about the size of my little finger that has about 400 calories. That's always good for energy."

Touring. "I always pack a trail mix of peanuts, banana chips, and raisins for when I'm touring and in stage races. I also carry along all kinds of fruits because they're easy to carry and digest. Water and juices are important, too."

Here are some of Brent's favorite recipes.

Tout the Trout
Not high on carbohydrates but good protein with little fat and a spiritually perfect way to end the day after a weekend tour.

1 pan-dressed trout (about ½ pound)
1 tablespoon olive oil
½ lemon
    Preheat oven to 350°F.
1. Wash the fish with cold water to remove any film and leave fish feeling "squeaky clean." Brush olive oil on both sides of fish and lay in oiled pan.
2. Slice the lemon very thinly and lay the slices edge to edge over the entire fish.
3. Bake 20 to 30 minutes, depending on the size of the fish, or until the fish flakes easily with a fork. Squeeze the lemon slices over the trout at the table.

Yield: 1 serving

Tortizzas
This is a tasty and well-balanced combination of carbohydrates, protein and fats.

2 flour or corn tortillas

2 teaspoons butter

¼ cup homemade or jar spaghetti sauce with or without meat

½ cup of any of the following: chopped onion, sliced mushrooms, diced tomatoes, sprouts, shredded carrots, chopped green peppers, etc. If you like it, put it on!

½ cup shredded cheese: cheddar, Swiss, mozzarella, provolone, etc.

2 tablespoons grated Parmesan cheese

oregano or Italian seasoning to taste

Preheat over to 350°F.

1. Spread 1 teaspoon butter on each tortilla, mainly near edges.

2. Spread 2 tablespoons sauce evenly on tortilla.

3. Mix vegetable ingredients and sprinkle over each tortilla to within ¼ inch of edge. Top with cheeses and oregano.

4. Bake on a lightly oiled cookie sheet for 10 to 15 minutes, depending on number of toppings.

Yield: 2 Tortizzas—1 biker-sized snack

Rice, Raisins and Sucrose

For use as quick energy meal (97 grams of carbohydrate per serving).

1 cup long-grain white rice

2 cups water

½ teaspoon salt

1 cup milk

¾ cup raisins

¼ cup sugar or 2 tablespoons honey

1. In a large saucepan combine rice, water, and salt. Bring to boil over high heat.

2. Reduce heat to simmer (low), cover pan and cook 12 to 14 minutes, or until water is absorbed.

3. Fluff with fork and allow to sit covered and off heat for 5 minutes.
4. Stir in milk, raisins, and sugar or honey.
5. Place in 3 two-cup bowls, cover and refrigerate overnight.

*Yield: 3 racer servings for criteriums or
tours or 1 stage-race-sized breakfast*

Your Liquid Needs. The most important thing you can carry in your water bottle is water. This vital fluid replenishes your sweat losses, transports oxygen and wastes to various sites in the body and prevents heat-related illnesses. Researchers have determined that 50°F to 55°F is the ideal temperature for water while exercising, as cool water leaves the stomach and is available to the body more quickly than tepid. Just don't drink *cold* water as it can cause stomach spasms.

A good rule of thumb is *drink before you have to*. If you wait until you feel thirsty, you're already well on the way to dehydration. According to Alan Strizak, Director of the Laboratory for the Evaluation of Achievement in Performance (LEAP) in Long Beach, California, "Our thirst mechanism isn't very sensitive so we need to keep up our fluid intake during cycling."

David Costill, Ph.D., a reknowned physiologist, agrees. In his laboratory at Ball State University, he's spent years studying the influence of fluid intake on both the long-distance runners and cyclists. While on sabbatical in Norway a few years ago, Costill had the opportunity to observe endurance cycling firsthand during the Trondheim–Oslo race, a 384-mile event whose nickname is "The Great Endurance Test." During the long event, the hardy cyclists were forced to eat and drink frequently to keep up their strength. As a result, Costill saw that the intake of fluids can be made difficult by a stomach full of food. "And even in our earlier laboratory studies, we've seen that even without eating solid foods, regulating fluid intake can be tricky during heavy exercise because the stomach sometimes does not empty fast enough to keep up with the very high rate of water being lost as sweat." His conclusion? "Force yourself to drink fluids as frequently as possible, even when your stomach feels 'full.'"

Some cyclists prefer a slightly sweetened liquid solution to just plain water. That's all right, providing the drink doesn't contain more than 2 to 2½ percent sugar. (Many commercial colas and fruit juices contain much more.)

In fact, many commercial drinks contain too much sugar (at least 10 percent) for the cyclist's body to process. "Strong sugar solutions draw fluids away from other parts of the body to the intestines," explains Daniel Hanley, Sr., M.D., head physician at Bowdoin College, "and as the solution passes through the [stomach and] digestive tract, it can create the need for an extra bowel movement. More dilute solutions (of 2 to 2½ percent) are an advantage to the cyclist, because they can be absorbed more rapidly in the bloodstream."

In other words, your goal in cycling is to get water circulating through the body as quickly as possible. It's best to avoid highly sugared drinks such as Kool-Aid and soft drinks that prevent this. Even some of the athletic drinks—Gatorade, for example—contain twice as much sugar as recommended. But you can dilute it.

If you're fond of these "thirst quenchers," don't despair. There are two athletic drinks, Pripps-Plus and Excel, which boast higher than normal concentrations of sugar, yet are not considered harmful to the cyclist. The reason is that the manufacturers have altered the carbohydrate's molecular structure, resulting in a drink that is highly concentrated with large particles of sugar that do not hamper the emptying of fluids from the stomach.

Still other manufacturers are investigating ways to reduce their products' overall sugar content. One suggestion for cyclists is to become an avid label reader to find out the sugar content for each product.

Another is to make your own "bike-ade." Here's one formula from Dr. Smith.

In a two-quart plastic or glass (not metal) container mix the following:

¼ cup sugar

½ teaspoon table salt

one package unsweetened Kool-Aid, for flavor (optional)

Add water to total two quarts. Fills four water bottles.

The ½ cup of sugar is one-fourth as much sugar as the Kool-Aid package calls for, but produces adequate sweetness. Diabetics and those on calorie-restricted diets will need to include the sugar in their calculated daily intake. The drink has about 100 calories per pint. The ½ teaspoon of salt tastes rather unpleasant in the kitchen, but seems okay on the road. (Those on low-salt diets or with high blood pressure should not add salt to their bike-ade.)

To make dehydrated bike-ade, to carry along on a long tour and add water as you go, make up the above mixture in a dry container with a tight-fitting top. Shake it up well, then divide into four equal portions, each of which is sealed in an envelope or plastic bag of some sort. Add one envelope to an empty pint-sized water bottle before refilling. The liquid mixture is best kept refrigerated, but this is not necessary for the powder.

To stretch the mix out, so that it lasts longer, carry at least two water bottles. Keep plain water in one, which you can use to douse your head and shoulders when it is really hot. Keep bike-ade in the other to drink.

The Salt Question. While water is the best substance to use to quench thirst or to sprinkle on your head for heat relief, it doesn't supply enough or replace electrolytes. An electrolyte (found in both sweat and in blood plasma) is a salt which, in a water solution, has lost one of its electrons.

For example, sodium is a positive ion because it has 11 positive charges and ten negative charges. It is a $+1$ charged ion.

Various studies have analyzed electrolyte levels in subjects before and after exercise to determine how much of each electrolyte is lost with heavy sweating.

We now know that for most cyclists, sodium and chloride losses are proportionately greater than other electrolyte deficits. Sodium and chloride, of course, make up that familiar commodity we know as salt.

Now there has been a lot of contradictory advice in recent years about salt for athletes. Here are some guidelines.

Don't take salt pills without water, as some athletes are inclined to do. The effect is just what you don't want: drawing water from the tissues to neutralize the salt you just dumped in, pushing you further along toward dehydration.

But it appears that exercise performance in the heat can be improved by the addition of minimal amounts of salt in your water bottle. Hence, the inclusion of salt in our homemade bike-ade.

One study which supports this conclusion took place in the desert where subjects drank as they walked for two hours. They had been divided into four groups to measure the effects of two variables. When the temperatures, heart rates, weight losses, sweat rates, and the chloride concentration in their sweat were compared, the group which fared best were those who drank cold water with a bit of salt added to it (a 0.1 percent saline solution). These investigators concluded that the higher weight loss experienced by those who drank pure water was due to salt depletion (*Journal of Applied Physiology*, Vol. 35, pp. 231–235, 1973).

A comprehensive review of other studies on salt losses substantiates those findings. So, of the various electrolytes present in prepared athletic drinks, sodium and chloride (salt) are the most important. If you're planning a long day on your bike in the heat and you want to duplicate drinks less expensively, try dropping one-quarter teaspoon of iodized salt or a half-gram salt tablet into your pint water bottle for an optimum electrolyte replacement drink. The salt taste is not obvious.

Riders most likely to benefit from this sort of salt replacement are those spinning in the heat for several hours a day, a few days in a row. Also it should help those cyclists who must suddenly ride in heat without having had the time to acclimatize. One important way our bodies acclimate to heat is that they begin to sweat more. Sweat becomes more dilute, and not so many electrolytes are lost. But that takes time.

Suffering in the heat is no joke for cyclists. Some try to compensate for sweat losses by going overboard. John Howard, the former "Ironman" who placed second in the 1982 Great American Bike Race, wilted under the oppressive desert sun. In an attempt to revive himself, he drank a potent mixture of water spiked with dolomite and potassium—the combination of which contributed to his nausea and fatigue. (In fact, scientists suggest the best way to replace potassium losses on long rides is simply snacking on bananas and oranges, standard cycling fare.)

Beating the Heat. When riding in the heat for several days, dehydration becomes a matter for concern. The best way to guard against dehydration is to check your weight every morning before breakfast. If you notice a two- to three-pound loss in body weight from morning to morning, you must increase your fluid intake. You need not worry about drinking too much, because your kidneys will unload the excess water in a matter of a few hours.

Here are a few other tips for cyclists to follow while riding in hot weather:

• Drink several ounces (8–10) of fluid 10 to 15 minutes before starting out.

• Drink several ounces of fluid from your water bottle every few miles. Don't wait until you are thirsty.

• Drinks should be low in sugar. A cool drink (45–55°F.) will also help in stomach emptying and aid in lowering body temperature.

• Be conscious of temperature and humidity conditions. A high percentage of humidity retards the evaporation of sweat from the skin.

• When warm weather begins, moderate your activity until acclimatized. Avoid exercising during the hottest part of the day.

• On a warm day wear light-colored, lightweight clothing that breathes. Don't ever wear extra layers or such instruments of torture as a vinyl jacket for the purpose of losing weight. All you lose is water, and the weight just goes back on when you drink.

• If you are overweight, your body is already working extra hard in the heat because you have more "insulation."

• Be familiar with the early warning symptoms of heat illness. *Early warning symptoms include: dizziness, grogginess, dry skin, rapid heart rate, chilling, nausea, unsteadiness, and throbbing in the head.* (Dizziness is almost always the first perceptible symptom. No need to panic; just stop, consume liquids if available, and rest for a while.)

Dairy Products.   One liquid that stirs up quite a controversy is milk. Some cyclists say it's good for them, citing Olympic cyclist Brent Emery's admission he drinks milk "by the quart." Others complain of "cotton-mouth" and stomach cramps whenever they imbibe and try to ride.

What's the truth about milk and the cyclist? In milk from cows, the carbohydrate lactose, known as "milk sugar," makes up four to five percent of the milk's total weight. A lactose molecule is made up of two substances, glucose and galactose, linked together. For your body to digest them, they must be split through hydrolysis, a process in which water combines with them. When all goes well, this takes place in a portion of the small intestine, facilitated by an enzyme called lactase. Lactase helps us digest lactose. But not everyone has a sufficient supply (or any at all) of the enzyme lactase to digest milk properly.

The problem occurs in varying degrees among different ethnic groups and in different parts of the world. For example, only about one or two percent of the Scandinavian population is affected, compared to 99 to 100 percent of Orientals. Generally speaking, the only people who can properly digest lactose are the cultural groups which have traditionally raised cattle and drunk milk—mostly Caucasians living in northern and western Europe and their descendents in other countries like ours. The problem exists but is relatively rare among this group. There is a high incidence of lactase deficiency among blacks, Orientals, Jews, and Native Americans in the United States.

What does a lactase deficiency mean to the intestines? If lactose cannot be hydrolyzed, it draws water by osmosis from the walls of the large intestine, is attacked by the bacteria which normally live there, and is made to ferment. All this can cause cramps, bloating, gas, and diarrhea; not pleasant, especially if it hits when you're out on the bike.

If you suffer from these symptoms and suspect you have a lactase deficiency, the first step is to keep a food diary. If there are recurring problems each time one eats milk products or drinks milk, the diary provides a valuable record. The next step would be experimenting by cutting down on or eliminating foods which contain lactose. With prepared foods, it may be necessary to read labels to be certain that the ingredients do not include milk or milk products. Again, record the results. If you suspect a lactase deficiency, consult your doctor.

Some physicians administer a lactose tolerance test in which, for adults, 50 grams of lactose, the amount in one quart of milk, are taken by mouth and then periodically blood samples are taken and the blood sugar level is measured. If you have plenty of the enzyme lactase, a marked increase in blood sugar should be observed. Conversely, low blood sugar levels point to a lactase deficiency.

Diagnosis of a lactase deficiency doesn't necessarily mean the end of eating all milk products. There are alternatives to milk, including cheeses such as Gouda and Edam which contain no lactose after ripening.

Fermented milk products like buttermilk, high-quality yogurt, and kefir can be tolerated more easily than liquid milk because the bacterial action in the starter culture alters some of the lactose. However, not just any supermarket yogurt will do. Avoid the Swiss-style yogurts altogether, and look for the words "contains active cultures," such as you'll see on the Colombo yogurt carton. The key word is "contains," since most yogurts are made with live cultures but some are heat-treated afterward for longer shelf-life. This kills the starter bacteria which appear to be beneficial to the lactase-deficient person. Dannon's labeling is more ambiguous, but it, too, is among the quality brands which still contain viable cultures.

Another way to avoid the troubles that go along with lactase intolerance is with an enzyme product called Lact-Aid, which is available in supermarkets and drug stores. Add a little packet of it to a quart of milk, and the enzyme, which comes from yeast, breaks down the lactose in the milk. Some dairies are now pretreating milk with this product; labeling on the carton will indicate when this is the case.

Fats and Sugar: A Word of Caution. While cyclists may include many dairy products, including milk (providing they're not lactase-deficient), cheese, yogurt, and ice cream in their *daily* diet, it is generally agreed these foods may not be suitable for endurance cycling.

The reason is that dairy products, while high in protein, also contain plenty of fat, particularly in the case of cheese and ice cream. High-fat foods take a long time to digest— several hours longer than quickly digested high-carbohydrate snacks.

"We'd never recommend to anyone the idea of eating ice cream while bicycling 100 miles," pointed out a nutritionist from Penn State University. "The digestive process is just too slow—emptying the stomach and intestinal contents can take anywhere from four to five hours."

Moreover, high-fat foods pose another drawback: Unlike carbohydrates, fats can not be metabolized into immediately usable muscle fuel. "Fat is not utilized as energy in the form in which it goes into the bloodstream after eating," points out Dr. Julian Whitaker, Director, California Heart Treatment Center. "Fat has to go through a long metabolic process."

"In order to utilize fat stores for fuel while exercising," he continues, "the cyclist needs to draw on his free fatty acid supply. Free fatty acids are broken down from fatty foods over a period of time. While touring or racing, cyclists won't derive any energy at all from a high-fat meal prior to exercise. Instead, they'll be drawing on fatty acid stores they've been training their bodies for weeks ahead of time to use."

For example, it is thought that with training the cyclist actually increases the number of capillary blood vessels which carry oxygen and fatty acids to the muscles. With a greater circulation of oxygen, fats can be burned more readily.

So burning fat efficiently as fuel becomes easier over

time with training—particularly by riding long hours. But many people don't understand that. A friend of mine boasts she eats high-fat foods like ice cream over lunch hour and then burns off the fat calories cycling home from work. I tried to explain that that was unlikely. She didn't care. "Listen," she added, "if it tastes good and works for me, why not?" (My friend has since gained five pounds.)

Of more consequence to the cyclist than the fat content of ice cream is its sugar content. Ice cream contains lots of sugar; in fact, one-eighth of a quart has about six teaspoons of sugar. Tests conducted at Ball State University have shown that ingesting a large amount of sugar just prior to a race can slow an athlete down and suggest it's best not to eat ice cream and then jump on your bike. Most researchers who have studied the subject agree.

When the cyclist eats a highly sugared food, large amounts of sugar are absorbed into the bloodstream. Large amounts of sugar also stimulate the release of insulin from the pancreas. This release of insulin, coupled with muscular activity at the start of the race, can cause the blood glucose level to fall rapidly during the first five or ten minutes of exercise, the very time when you need all your juices flowing. At Ball State, subjects grew fatigued earlier and found running more difficult when they took a sugared drink 30 to 45 minutes before the race.

However, once you start exercising and get over that initial hump, you can eat slightly sugared substances, at least to a degree. The release of insulin by the pancreas is suppressed once exercise is started. However, candy bars and other highly sugared foods still cause havoc.

So the rule of thumb concerning ice cream is: No cones up to two hours before riding because of the sugar content; and no ice cream while riding if you don't think your body can handle the fat content. Whether all that ice cream fat will sit comfortably in your stomach during leisurely cycling varies greatly with the individual.

While ice cream seems to top most riders' "favorites" list, there *are* other frozen alternatives. Ice milk, for instance, has about one-third of the fat that's in ice cream. That may appeal to cyclists concerned about fat sitting in their stomachs. The only catch, however, is that ice milk and even soft ice cream have more sugar than regular ice cream. The sugar adds weight and texture to compensate for less milk fat.

Frozen yogurt, considered by many as an appealing change from ice cream, has some drawbacks too. Although the dietary delight has less cholesterol and fat than ice cream, it can contain a large amount of sugar.

Of course, no one's suggesting you give up ice cream completely. After all, there are things that just can't be sacrificed; as Don Kaidong, a world-class marathoner, once pointed out, "Without ice cream, there would be chaos and darkness in the world."

Beer. Any discussion of fluids would have to conclude with a popular yet controversial cycling beverage: alcohol.

Some cyclists, particularly during long rides, enjoy stopping for a beer, a practice which Ed Burke suggests won't be harmful. "The key is moderation," he insists. "A little alcohol is okay. But more than one or two beers can be dehydrating."

In effect, alcohol "turns off" the antidiuretic hormone from the pituitary gland that helps the body regulate and retain the water it needs. Cyclists who overindulge will find themselves urinating frequently and may even, in very hot weather, risk dehydration. The moral: It's probably safer not to ride and drink, but a small amount of alcohol won't hurt.

For many the real pleasure of a long ride or tour is to stop for a leisurely lunch or a long dinner and enjoy a couple of beers. I practice that ritual myself.

It's a small pleasure after cycling a hundred miles.

Recipes

Following are some on-the-road high energy snacks prepared by Anita Hirsch of the Rodale Press Food Kitchen, Kretschmer Wheat Germ products, and *Bicycling* magazine readers:

Energy Balls

½ cup raisins
2 tablespoons protein powder or soy flour
1 tablespoon nutritional yeast
½ cup wheat germ (raw)
½ cup sunflower seeds
1½ cups peanut butter
2 tablespoons molasses
⅓ cup honey
½ cup shredded coconut (unsweetened)

Soak the ½ cup raisins in a little water for about 10 minutes. Mix the soy flour and nutritional yeast in a large bowl with 3 tablespoons of the wheat germ. Add the sunflower seeds and raisins (drained of water they were soaking in). In another bowl stir together the peanut butter, molasses and honey. Fold this into the ingredients of the first bowl until the dry ingredients are absorbed and mixed well.

On a flat plate lightly mix the coconut and remaining wheat germ. Scoop a spoonful of the peanut butter mixture and roll in the coconut mixture shaping into a round ball as you roll (about 1½ inches). Continue same with rest. Makes about 16.

A banana can be added to the peanut butter mixture to

make a more moist, fluffy, good-tasting energy ball. These are not as suitable for traveling or unrefrigeration though.

Ann McCoy
Eureka, California

Great Balls O' Fire

1 cup carob chips
1 cup peanut butter
2 cups oatmeal

Melt carob chips in a pot over low heat. Stir constantly. Do not let chips burn. Remove when smooth. Add peanut butter and stir in mix completely. Add oatmeal. Stir until combined.

Roll in spoon-size balls and refrigerate till hardened. Keep in cool, dry place. Makes 30 balls about 1-inch diameter.

Karen LeMond
Carson City, Nevada

Carob-Nut Candy

1 cup honey
1 cup peanut butter
1 cup carob powder
1 cup sesame seeds, lightly toasted
2 cups shelled sunflower seeds
½ cup shredded unsweetened coconut
½ cup chopped dates, apricots or raisins

Butter an 8-inch square pan. Heat honey and peanut butter together in heavy saucepan. Quickly mix in all remaining ingredients. Spread into prepared pan and refrigerate about 2 hours, or until firm.

Cut into squares to serve. Store in refrigerator. Wrap individually in plastic when using on trips. Makes 5 dozen 1-inch squares.

Diane Hanke
Milwaukee, Wisconsin

Tahini Candy

2 tablespoons Tahini (sesame butter)
1 cup powdered milk (or any powdered grain)
¼ cup honey
½ cup finely chopped dates
⅓ cup carob powder
¼ teaspoon vanilla
2 teaspoons debittered Brewer's yeast

Mix all ingredients together with hands. Form into a roll or balls. Chill, but not necessary. Slice and coat with coconut, sesame seeds or nut meal. Makes 30 balls of approximately 1-inch diameter.

Maury McCullough
Tulsa, Oklahoma

Strawberry-Nut Bread

1 cup strawberries (or other fruit)
⅓ cup water
1¾ cups whole wheat flour
1 teaspoon baking soda
½ teaspoon cinnamon
½ cup honey
⅓ cup butter
2 eggs
½ cup chopped walnuts

Heat strawberries and water to boiling over medium heat and cook one minute, stirring constantly; cool, then purée.

Combine flour, baking soda and cinnamon in a large mixing bowl. Cream honey, butter and eggs until light and fluffy. Alternately add flour mixture and water to creamed mixture, mixing at low speed of electric mixer. Stir in puréed cooked strawberries. Fold in walnuts.

Spread batter in a greased 9″ x 5″ loaf pan and bake in a 350°F. oven for about one hour, or until toothpick inserted in center comes out clean.

Cool in pan ten minutes; remove from pan and cool completely on wire rack.

Mellow bread by wrapping with foil or plastic wrap and storing at room temperature for 24 hours, if desired. Makes one loaf.

Anita Hirsch

Blueberry-Cashew Bread

2 cups whole wheat flour
1½ teaspoons baking powder
½ teaspoon baking soda
1 cup broken pieces roasted, unsalted cashews
1 cup fresh blueberries
¾ cup buttermilk or yogurt
2 tablespoons oil
2 eggs
½ cup honey

Combine all ingredients. Mix until smooth and pour into greased 9″ x 5″ loaf pan and bake at 350°F. for 60 to 70 minutes.

Cool completely before removing from pan. Makes one loaf.

Anita Hirsch

Banana Orange Muffins

1½ cups whole wheat flour
2 teaspoons baking powder
⅛ teaspoon salt
1 cup wheat germ
1 tablespoon Brewer's yeast
1 cup mashed banana (2 medium bananas)
⅓ cup honey or molasses
½ cup orange juice
¼ cup cooking oil
2 eggs
½ cup raisins (optional)

Stir together dry ingredients. In separate bowl combine remaining ingredients. Pour liquids all at once into dry ingredients. Stir just until all ingredients are moistened. Do not overmix. Fill greased muffin pans. Bake at 400°F. for 20 to 25 minutes or until brown. Makes 12 muffins.

Jean M. Lown
Providence, Rhode Island

Cyclist's Squares

2 eggs, separated
2 tablespoons honey
⅓ cup safflower oil
1 cup whole wheat flour
¼ cup wheat germ
2 tablespoons soy flour
2 tablespoons rice flour
1 tablespoon Brewer's yeast
1 cup golden raisins
½ cup raw sunflower seeds
1 teaspoon vanilla

Beat egg yolks. Add honey gradually while beating yolks; then add oil. Mixture will be lumpy. Add whole wheat flour, wheat germ, soy flour, rice flour and Brewer's yeast. The mixture will be crumbly. Press into 13″ x 9″ greased pan. Beat egg whites until stiff and add raisins, sunflower seeds and vanilla.

Spread this mixture over flour mixture. Bake at 325°F. for 25 minutes or until brown. Cut into squares when cool. Makes 18.

Anita Hirsch

Rice Cakes

2½ cups cooked rice (1 cup raw)
¼ cup butter
2 tablespoons honey
4 eggs
½ teaspoon cinnamon
¼ teaspoon kelp
1 teaspoon grated lemon rind
½ cup seedless raisins (optional)

Cream butter and honey. Beat in eggs one at a time. Add remaining ingredients, including cooked rice.

Bake in a greased 8″ cake pan for one hour at 350°F. until brown. Cool, and then refrigerate. Cut into wedges and wrap for the road. Yield: 8 slices.

Anita Hirsch

Zucchini Bread

Preheat oven to 325°F.
  3 eggs
  1 cup honey
  2 teaspoons vanilla
  1 cup oil
  ¼ teaspoon baking powder
  1 teaspoon baking soda
  3½ teaspoons cinnamon
  2 cups whole wheat flour
  ¼ cup wheat germ
  ¼ cup bran
  2 cups grated zucchini, unpeeled
  ¾ cup chopped nuts
  ½ cup raisins, optional

Beat eggs and honey together. Stir in vanilla and oil. Combine dry ingredients and add to first mixture, beating well. Stir in zucchini, nuts and raisins. Pour into two greased loaf pans and bake at 325°F. for 60 to 70 minutes.

Cool in pans before serving. Makes two loaves. *Note:* this bread freezes very well.

Wheat Germ Granola

  3 cups rolled oats
  1½ cups wheat germ
  ½ cup chopped almonds
  ⅓ cup sesame seeds
  ¼ cup cooking oil
  ¼ cup honey
  1 cup raisins

Combine all ingredients *except* raisins, mixing well. Spread mixture evenly in large shallow pan. Bake at

300°F. for 30 minutes, stirring every 10 minutes, until lightly toasted. Stir in raisins. Cool.

Store covered in refrigerator. Makes 6½ to 7 cups.

Kretschmer Wheat Germ Products

Bicycle Energy Bars

½ cup basic carob syrup (See recipe below)
¼ cup honey
2 tablespoons butter
2 tablespoons peanut butter
¾ cup wheat germ
¾ cup rolled oats
½ cup flaked coconut
½ cup finely snipped pitted dates

In large saucepan over low heat combine carob syrup, honey, butter and peanut butter until melted. Add all remaining ingredients, mixing well. Shape quickly with buttered hands into eight bars, about 3 inches long. Wrap each bar in plastic wrap. Refrigerate until firm. Makes 8 bars.

Substitute dried apricots for the dates to make Apricot Bars.

Basic Carob Syrup

1 cup carob powder
1 cup water

In a small saucepan, mix carob and water. Bring to a boil over very low heat, stirring constantly. Cook for 5 to 8 minutes or until the syrup is completely smooth. Cool and store, covered, in refrigerator. Makes about 1½ cups.

Kretschmer Wheat Germ Products

Wholesome Muffins

3 eggs
½ cup oil
1½ cups milk
3 tablespoons honey
1 tablespoon pure vanilla
1 cup whole wheat flour
1 cup rolled oats
1 cup natural bran
½ cup wheat germ
2 tablespoons baking powder
½ teaspoon baking soda
1 cup sesame seeds
½ cup desiccated coconut
1 cup raisins
1 cup chopped dates

Beat together first five ingredients. Mix together all dry ingredients. Add liquid to the dry; mix until just moist. Bake at 375°F. for 20 minutes. Makes two dozen muffins.

Anita Hirsch
Rodale Press

Oven-Dried Beef Jerky (Charqui con Chile)

2 pounds boneless beef (chuck roast)
chili sauce (See recipe below)
black pepper

Slice the beef into ¼-inch thick strips. Marinate beef strips in chili sauce overnight. Drain beef, spread out on baking sheets and sprinkle with black pepper. Dry in oven at lowest temperature (120°F.) for 4 to 5 hours. Leave oven door slightly open for moisture to escape.

Homemade Chili Sauce

9 fresh green chili peppers (or 2 pounds dried chili pods
   or 1 package frozen red chilis)
1 teaspoon oregano
3½ cups water
½ teaspoon crushed cilantro (coriander)
1 clove crushed garlic
8-ounce can tomato sauce
2 tablespoons flour

Wash chili peppers, roast in oven at 350°F. for 15
minutes. (Dried chili only has to be toasted for two
minutes.) Remove stems and seeds from peppers. Do not
touch your hands to your eyes. Blend chili peppers
thoroughly in the blender with a little of the water.
Combine with other ingredients except flour, simmer for
15 minutes. Add flour to thicken sauce by sprinkling over
sauce while stirring.

Benny Sena
Las Animas, Colorado

14

Your Weight Loss Program

If I had a magic formula by which you could lose weight and keep it off, I'd be rich. I don't and I'm not.

So much absolute nonsense is being tossed around these days about losing weight while eating more, losing pounds while exercising less. It is a billion-dollar business getting fat on itself.

However, I do have a formula that's simple and unremarkable: regular cycling and sensible eating. As you will see in the "Weight Loss Stories" that appear throughout this chapter, regular cycling and sensible eating will take off the pounds—a lot of pounds. One man weighed 275 pounds and had a 46-inch waist. Daily cycling was a major factor in his losing 90 pounds. A woman, who had struggled for years to lose weight with miracle diets, discovered cycling was the real cure. She not only lost weight, she significantly improved her lean body mass.

In the first chapter I wrote about cycling being a lifesport, an activity you could stay with at your pace for the rest of your life. But cycling is more than an activity; it can be a way of life, as well as a way of exercise. If you cycle to lose weight, the context will soon change. Yes, your body's metabolism will speed up and you will likely lose pounds. But you are shedding pounds within a context of pleasure and independence. Quite likely the matter of weight loss will become a secondary item as you develop your endurance and sense of importance. If there is one thought that stays with me after talking to and corresponding with thousands of people who cycle to lose weight, it's that they take for granted weight loss or weight stabilization after they have embraced a strenuous cycling program.

I'm in the Pocono Mountains in northern Pennsylvania writing this chapter. I had eggs, lean sausage and toast for breakfast this morning, which I figure is about 600 calories. At lunchtime I went out for a long ride, maybe twenty miles, so I figure I used up most of those calories. I'm no different from anyone else. I like to count the calories coming in and going out. But if the significance of my riding stopped there, I would be very disappointed.

Because of the rough road and rocky terrain I'm riding an all-terrain bike called the Stump-Jumper. I was musing about the name, wondering whether the bike could really jump over a stump—it could in the hands of a better and more daring bike handler—when a deer leapt over both me and the bike. My heart racing, my first thought was editorial—was there a story here?—Believe It or Not, Deer Jumps Stump-Jumper.

During my ride I saw many deer along the ski trails, most darting out far ahead of my bike. The quiet here in the mountains, especially after the grunt and roar of city life, is awesome. Thanks to the fat tires on the all-terrain bike I was able to push far out into the skiing areas, deserted till the fall. The silence was so complete that I took my pulse. My body never sounded so loud.

A few years ago there was much talk about lightening the bike for competition. Some cyclists went to great lengths, including drilling holes in the cranks, just to eliminate a gram or two. While that mania appears to have subsided, there have been at least two generations of components which claim to be worth their weight in grams.

WEIGHT LOSS SUCCESS #1

Charles Bonetti of Portland, Maine, was 225 pounds and had a blood pressure reading of 130/90 and climbing. He was a heart attack waiting to happen. So he borrowed his daughter's three-speed and started cycling one or two miles a day. Within weeks he was up to 10–15 miles per trip. He began to lose ounces, then pounds and, feeling a real sense of accomplishment, increased the mileage.

For his 52nd birthday, his daughter bought him a 12-speed and his mileage increased dramatically. By the end of the summer he was riding 300–350 miles a week. Even in the winter he managed to cycle 25–30 miles a day on weekends. He uses an indoor exercise bike when he can't get outside. He is now cycling to work and back, which is 31 miles each way.

Indirectly, he credits cycling for his weight loss. "When you are biking," he writes, "you are burning calories and are more aware of proper eating habits."

He is now 53 and weighs 175 pounds, a drop of 50 pounds in a year. His blood pressure is 118/78 and his doctor finds him in excellent shape.

The cycling press has responded to this obsession with lightness by publishing cartoons showing every aspect of the bike drilled out, including the rider himself. The point: Taking weight off the rider probably makes more economic sense. If you wanted to decrease the total weight of your bike and components by, say, ten pounds, depending on what you are currently riding, it could cost a few hundred dollars. If you're riding a 38-pound mass-merchant special, you could trade that in for around $300 and walk away ten pounds lighter. A significant decrease in total bike weight after that would likely mean buying a bike well over $500.

What's more important, the weight you are sitting on or the weight that is sitting on you? No contest. Certainly you want a responsive, lightweight bike and the more you cycle the more important that fact will be—and you will adjust accordingly. But, in the long run, you will become a more efficient cyclist by losing those ten pounds wrapped around your waist.

WEIGHT LOSS SUCCESS #2

Gary C. Dolde of Chesapeake City, Maryland, knew that when the bottom figure on his blood pressure reading was over 100, he was in trouble. Though he didn't feel too bad, he knew that at five-eight he shouldn't weigh 210 pounds and sport a 38-inch waist. By the time he conferred with his doctor, his weight was 214 pounds. His physician put him on medication and a weight reduction diet.

Knowing that if he stayed around the house he would be hard put to ignore food, he started cycling, five miles a day the first week, then ten. He lost four pounds the first week.

He set stiffer goals for himself. How quickly could he do ten miles? In 30 minutes? He increased his mileage to 20, 25 and 50 miles, the latter with a local club.

Six months later he discontinued the blood pressure medicine as his weight was down to 175 pounds.

If you are overweight, you're in the company of 30 percent of Americans who are considered heavy by normal standards. And that includes many recreational cyclists who ride only a few times a year.

No one has to tell you if you're overweight. A glance in the mirror is usually sufficient. Norman Sheil, former coach of the British and Canadian Olympic cycling teams, suggests you "Try a simple pinch test at waist level just above and to the rear of your hips. This should tell you all you need to know to lose weight."

Dieters traditionally consult the weight/height charts published by life insurance companies and broadcast in the popular press. As noted in an earlier chapter, these charts can be misleading. Far more important than your total weight is what percentage of your body is fat and what percentage is lean body mass (bone, muscle, and water). As you age, if you don't exercise and watch your diet, you will see a proportionate decrease in your lean body mass, even if you manage to maintain the same weight in your 50s you enjoyed in your 20s.

While your honest bathroom scale will give you a reliable reading of your total weight, it won't tell you much about your body fat. The best way to determine that is with a pair of calipers once for the exclusive use of physicians and researchers but now available to the rest of us through medical supply outlets and pharmacies. By all means ask your physician how to use them. Simply, the calipers measure skin and fat as it's pulled from muscle, usually at biceps, triceps, below the shoulder blade and above the hip.

To accurately take skinfold measurements you will need the help of another person. Use a standard fat caliper available at hospital supply stores for the best results. Otherwise, you can use a small, hand-controlled pressure caliper purchased at a craft or hardware store, with readings measured against a millimeter scale or an ordinary ruler.

In taking measurements the thumb and forefinger of one hand are used to pinch and lift the skin and fat tissue away from the muscle. Two readings should be taken, preferably in the morning. At the hip pick up a skinfold halfway between the lower rib and hipbone, in a vertical line from the armpit. At the triceps, with the arm alongside the body, pick up the skinfold between the elbow and armpit. For the biceps measurement use the same methods. For a measurement at the shoulder blade pick up a skinfold below the blade itself.

The accompanying chart shows body fat content as the sum of the measurement of skinfolds at four sites. While skinfold measurement is not a difficult task, if you are uncertain of the procedure, get some help from your physician or at your local YMCA or health club.

If you are male, you'll want to aim for about 15 percent total body fat; a woman, about 22 percent. You might like to know that when the U.S. National Cycling Team was measured a few years ago, the women had an average of 15.4 percent body fat and men 8.8 percent.

As you become more fit and look for more exquisite measurements of your weight and well-being, take a tip from Jacques Boyer, whom you have met before. Boyer thinks weight on the legs is an important clue and suggests, "You look for fat layers on your legs by pinching the skin with your fingers. If you're in shape, you just have a thin layer of skin over your legs, and the skin is very loose. If you do this often enough, you can begin to tell the fluctuations."

TABLE FIFTEEN

BODY FAT

Total Skin Fold (mm)	Men	Women	Boys	Girls
15	5.5	—	9.0	12.5
20	9.0	15.5	12.5	16.0
25	11.5	18.5	15.5	19.0
30	13.5	21.0	17.5	21.5
35	15.5	23.0	19.5	23.5
40	17.0	24.5	21.5	25.0
45	18.5	26.0	23.0	27.0
50	20.0	27.5	24.0	28.5
55	21.0	29.0	25.5	29.5
60	22.0	30.0	26.5	30.5
65	23.0	31.0	27.5	32.0
70	24.0	32.5	28.5	33.0
75	25.0	33.5	29.5	34.0
80	26.0	34.0		
85	26.5	35.0		
90	27.5	36.0		
95	28.0	36.5		

Reprinted with permission by professors Durin and Womersley, Institute of Physiology, The University of Glasgow, Scotland.

WEIGHT LOSS SUCCESS #3

At 28, D. M. Anderson of Santa Rosa, California, was 40 pounds overweight. He decided to do something about it and started cycling to work, seven miles away. On the first day the return trip took him an hour and a half. He could hardly breathe or walk when he arrived.

> The fact that he had been smoking for 16 years made cycling very difficult, so he had to make a choice. He threw his cigarettes in the garbage can and struggled with withdrawal symptoms for weeks.
>
> That was 12 years ago. The 40 pounds have not returned, nor have the cigarettes.

Getting Started. You've probably already had your fill of authorities who promote a variety of diets from protein supplements to carrot juice for weight loss—and I won't go into them here. The only way to lose weight and keep it off is by regular exercise and sensible eating. In a way a commitment to weight loss is a life-style change. You will have to modify the habits and ingredients that caused the problem in the first place.

While you might begin cycling to lose weight, that needn't be your preoccupation in the beginning. You've already learned how to begin your program with an eye to getting your legs and lungs in shape. Clinical evidence indicates that the more you exercise, the easier it is to lose weight. Studies conducted by Michael Pollock, Ph.D., director of the Human Performance Laboratory at the Mt. Sinai Hospital in Milwaukee, Wisconsin, confirm this. The men and women who exercised three or more times a week and cut back on calories lost both body fat and weight. Those who restricted their diets and exercised once or twice a week lost neither. Pollock concluded that, "We see the best results when you exercise three or more times a week."

Exercising every other day offers other benefits, including appetite suppression. According to William Fink, an associate professor at Ball State University, "Those who do not exercise at all usually are hungrier than those who exercise to a moderate degree. And those who exercise strenuously are hungrier than those who exercised moderately. Somehow moderate exercise depresses the appetite to a small degree.

"This appetite suppressing effect seems to be related to your activity level. Most people who run two miles (or cycle the equivalent) will probably find their appetite slightly depressed."

If moderate cycling suppresses your appetite, it also has a salutary effect on your *basal metabolic rate* (BMR), the rate at which your body burns up energy during its resting state. Although your BMR is influenced by many factors—age, weight, and sex among them—the Food and Nutrition Board estimates that the average adult male (154 pounds) burns between 1,440–1,728 calories a day. The average female (128 pounds) burns between 1,296–1,584 calories for basic metabolism.

Importantly, these figures will increase when you begin your cycling program. Vigorous cycling will burn up calories but will also increase your BMR for many hours after the actual exercise has ceased.

Riding for a half hour or an hour, for example, will stimulate the thyroid gland to produce a substance called thyroxin. Along with the adrenalines produced by the adrenal glands, thyroxin increases metabolic activity during exercise and, though to a lesser extent, for hours afterward. Exercise is like money that never stops earning interest, since it's possible to have as much as a 25-percent increase in basal metabolism for 15 hours after the exercise is over. As a cyclist, you'll be burning many more calories during the day, *even while at rest*, than you did in your previous life-style.

The various training programs already outlined will help you organize your weight loss program. Just because you have a lot of weight to lose you shouldn't try to speed up the process. If you haven't cycled for years, it will take some time for you to become acclimated to the bike. Don't jeopardize your program by becoming too ambitious in the beginning. Again, your first consideration should be position and form, no matter how difficult they might seem. Concentrate on your cadence and style. Get your rpm up to around 90. Get in your base mileage. Balance your hard and easy days.

For weight loss, I advise cycling moderately for periods up to an hour or more, three or four times a week. By this point in your training you no longer equate pushing down on the pedals with fitness; you equate spinning in a comfortable gear with high-performance cycling. That is the key to weight loss.

WEIGHT LOSS SUCCESS #4

The last exercise John Silvernail of St. Louis, Missouri, recalls getting was when he was in the Navy—and that was 23 years ago. At age 47 he was 245 pounds on a six-one frame. He could hardly bend to tie his shoelaces.

Though he started a diet and lost some weight he knew he would gain back the pounds if he didn't exercise. So he purchased a $250 bike and on his first ride experienced genuine agony.

After he had conditioned his rear end, back and legs, he began doing one-hour sprints at 75 percent of his natural heart rate. He joined a cycling club for tours, and rides at least 100 miles a week. He works out 30–45 minutes a day, five days a week and eats just about anything he wants to.

He has upgraded himself and his bike. In less than a year he lost 60 pounds. He also purchased a $600 Trek and a Turbo-Trainer for exercising indoors.

How do you distinguish between loafing and exercising on a bike? By now your legs should be delivering that distinction loud and clear. A consistently reliable guide to the strenuousness of your workout is your Training Heart Rate. I invite you to review the formula in Chapter Seven.

Checking Your Pulse.   You should get in the habit of taking your resting pulse at the wrist on waking each morning. Take a full one-minute count. Track this for a number of mornings in a row as there could be fluctuations.

I have found that it is very educational to stop and take my pulse from time-to-time during the day. I have a very obvious vein at my left wrist. When I want to check my pulse, I just look down and can get a fairly good idea of my heart rate. I have made the mistake of getting my pulse "read" by one of those machines popping up in drug stores across the nation. My pulse and blood pressure were so high that I immediately called my doctor. Later I learned about how inaccurate these machines can be.

Taking your exercise pulse is a little trickier, but when you are comfortable riding one-handed, you can take a pulse at your neck while coasting. Press your neck very lightly—to feel the pulsations with your fingers. Take the pulse for six seconds only, then multiply by ten to arrive at your rate per minute. You may find it easier to mount your watch on your handlebars to do this. There are also several cycling computers which you can hook up to your bike to keep track of your heart rate as you ride.

It also really helps to have a cycling log—in which you keep track of daily, weekly, and monthly mileage or time on the bike. It's surprising how that little log book becomes a conscience to help you get you out the door on days when you need encouragement.

Counting Your Losses.   A cycling log, also known as a training diary, can help you keep tabs on your daily diet too. While regular cycling is crucial to weight loss, so is a sensible weekly menu. Logging the foods you eat daily (and their calorie equivalent) will keep you honest.

Basically, dieting is a matter of mathematics. Every pound of body fat equals 3,500 calories. To lose one pound a week, you must reduce your caloric intake by 500 each day; bicycle (or do a similar aerobic sport) for at least an hour daily to burn up 500 calories; or both restrict your diet and increase your exercise to equal the expenditure of 3,500 calories over a week's time. For example, an hour's leisurely stroll burns up 200 calories. Step up the pace, and you can burn about 300. Now alter your diet slightly by skipping the teaspoons of sugar that usually accompany your coffee and substitute an apple for ice cream for dessert to save a total of about 200 calories. In all, by very simple steps you've managed to eliminate up to 500 calories in the course of the day.

It is often very difficult to determine *exactly* how many calories you burn while cycling, as speed, cadence and even the terrain determine caloric expenditure. Those cycling computers which measure your heart rate which we mentioned above also determine your cadence and speed, so if you're really serious about keeping an accurate calorie count, you'll want to invest in one.

David L. Smith, M.D., medical correspondent for *Bicycling* magazine, has devised a chart which provides a reasonable rule of thumb for you to determine your caloric expenditure, based on horsepower output and terrain. In the higher range, some of these figures are a little fanciful but Dr. Smith has included them to show us what isn't possible. When trying to lose weight through cycling you should attempt the possible.

TABLE SIXTEEN

HORSEPOWER OUTPUT
Crouched Cyclist on a Reasonably Efficient Bicycle

175-Pound Combination*

		Forward Speed (mph, assuming no wind)				
		10	15	20	25	30
Percent Grade	−2	coasting	coasting	.0399	.1743	.3918
	0	.0468	.1118	.2265	.4076	.6718
	+2	.1402	.2518	.4132	.641	.9518
	+5	.2802	.4618	.6932	.991	1.3718

200-Pound Combination

		Forward Speed (mph, assuming no wind)				
		10	15	20	25	30
Percent Grade	−2	coasting	coasting	.0203	.498	.3624
	0	.0504	.1171	.2336	.4165	.6824
	+2	.1571	.2771	.4469	.6832	1.0024
	+5	.3171	.5171	.7669	1.0832	1.4824

*Weight of cyclist plus bicycle

TABLE SEVENTEEN

CALORIE CONSUMPTION

175-Pound Combination*

		Forward Speed (mph, assuming no wind)				
		10	15	20	25	30
Percent Grade	−2	none	none	107	470	1057
	0	126	301	611	1100	1813
	+2	379	680	1116	1631	2570
	+5	757	1247	1872	2676	3704

200-Pound Combination

		Forward Speed (mph, assuming no wind)				
		10	15	20	25	30
Percent Grade	−2	none	none	55	404	978
	0	136	316	631	1124	1842
	+2	424	748	1207	1845	2706
	+5	856	1396	2071	2925	4003

*Weight of cyclist plus bicycle

WEIGHT LOSS SUCCESS #5

Edward Crawley of Massapequa, New York, had a heart attack when he was 37. He was 275 pounds, five-eleven, with a 46-inch waist. His blood pressure was 140/90.

Six years later he decided to diet and exercise, purchasing a Panasonic 12-speed and a Tunturi Ergometer for indoor use. He gradually worked up to 20 miles a day (10 miles inside during bad weather).

Seven years after, he weighs 185 pounds with a 37-inch waist. He has a resting pulse of 58 and a blood pressure reading of 110/70. He is no longer on medication.

Determining weight loss from cycling is not always an absolute science because the fitter you get, the slower you burn calories, which is really a function of heart rate. The heart of an unfit person beats faster than the heart of a trained individual. When the unfit person exercises he has to work harder.

The following chart published by *The Fitness Institute Bulletin* shows the number of calories you would burn a minute at various training heart rates, depending on how fit you are. For example, if you cycled 10 minutes at a heart rate of 180, you would burn about 90 calories. But if you were in top condition you might only expend 70 calories for the same effort.

TABLE EIGHTEEN

CALORIES PER MINUTE BASED ON EXERCISE HEART RATE AND FITNESS LEVEL

Heart Rate/Minute							
180	9.0	11.0	13.0	14.5	16.0	17.5	19.0
170	8.4	10.1	12.0	13.3	14.8	16.1	17.5
160	7.7	9.2	11.0	12.2	13.5	14.8	16.0
150	7.0	8.3	9.9	11.1	12.3	13.3	14.5
140	6.4	7.4	8.8	10.0	11.0	12.0	13.0
130	5.7	6.5	7.7	8.9	9.8	10.6	11.5
120	5.0	5.6	6.6	7.7	8.5	9.2	10.0
110	4.3	4.7	5.5	6.5	7.2	7.9	8.5
100	3.6	3.8	4.4	5.3	6.0	6.5	7.0
	Very Poor	Poor	Fair	Good	Very Good	Excellent	Superior

FITNESS CATEGORY

I caution you against playing the numbers game and applying any of these figures in absolute terms. We are all different, metabolically speaking. Our bodies respond to exercise and foods in different ways. I can usually get away with a couple of extra beers on a weekend, but should my wife be tempted by that extra piece of cake and ice cream she pays the price on Monday.

You should know that mile for mile, when practiced strenuously enough, cycling will burn up as many calories as any other activity. You can lose weight by cycling. But how much you lose and over what period of time will depend on how faithful you are to the program and your own metabolism. If the subjects cited in this chapter's success stories can lose weight, so can you.

WEIGHT LOSS SUCCESS #6

When he returned from the Vietnam War, Randall W. Brown weighed 178 pounds on a six-foot frame. Thirteen years later he weighed 272 pounds and suffered from high blood pressure and hypertension.

He mapped out a three-year fitness plan. The first year he rode a bike three miles, three days a week, walked a lot, ate only salads, fruits and vegetables—and lost 53 pounds. A year later he purchased a 12-speed and rode to work daily and put in longer rides in the evenings and on weekends. Within two months he lost another 18 pounds.

He is closing in on his goal: 185 pounds.

Consider the story of Paul McLeod, 30, of Cypress, California, who, tipping the scales at 242—on a six-foot frame—decided to lose weight the hard way: on a stationary bike in a college sports lab under the watchful eye of his instructor, who put him on a five-days-a-week exercise schedule. He also cut back on his calories.

Using a Monark Ergometer, common in sports labs or YMCAs, he cycled the first week at a torque (resistance) of 2 for 30 consecutive minutes at a 25-kilometer-per-hour rate. On the first day he burned 275.5 calories and the lab tested his lung capacity at about 6.8 liters of oxygen per minute. Within a month he had increased the torque force to 3, his oxygen intake to 10 liters a minute, and his caloric burn to 361. And he lost 14 pounds.

Within four months McLeod lost 40 pounds. His average 30-minute ride was 12.5 km during which be burned 500 calories and doubled his oxygen uptake rate.

During the second year of the program he reduced his weight to around 186. He acknowledges trying rapid weight loss programs. He writes: "As a high school wrestler I dropped 18 pounds in three days to make weight at a tournament. I ballooned from 205 to 225 as a freshman in college, then cut back to 185 over a three-month period on a steady diet of Coca-Cola and salads."

Does he find riding a stationary bike boring? Not at all; he "devours a pair of major metropolitan dailies each ride." If that is not your choice, he suggests watching television or listening to contemporary music, the kind that makes you work.

Does he find it work? Of course, but "losing weight was not intended to be a cakewalk."

McLeod concludes that the "ergometer has changed my life without drastically altering my life-style. As a baby boomer in the era of the echo effect, I want my two-year-old daughter to realize the pitfalls of sedentary labor, the meaning of proper health care and the methods available of balancing the two."

While it is sometimes tricky to figure out how many calories you burn while riding, it's easy to figure how many calories you're taking *in* at the dinner table. You can buy a booklet that lists many foods and their caloric equivalent at grocery stores or write to the United States Department of Agriculture for more information.

If the idea of keeping a running tally on what you eat doesn't thrill you, this should: *By our estimates, you can lose two pounds a week simply by regular bicycling, eating a balanced diet and restricting your intake of sweets*. Choose a good selection of foods from the four basic groups, including two servings of a meat, fish or other protein; four or more servings of breads, grains and cereals; four or more servings of fruits and vegetables; and two servings of milk and dairy products.

It's especially important to eat plenty of complex carbohydrates—foods such as breads, pastas, dried legumes and grain dishes. No matter what you've heard about the benefits of high-protein diets, nutritionists now say carbohydrates should be the mainstay of any weight-loss program. In fact, complex carbohydrates were the only food group which the Senate Select Committee on Nutrition and Human Needs recommended in the late 1970s that Americans should eat *more* of. That advice still holds true today.

The reason? Gram per gram, carbohydrates have less than *half* the calories of fat, yet provide valuable nutrients, vitamins and minerals.

But not all carbohydrates are good for you. While complex carbohydrates receive high marks, eating lots of simple carbohydrates (sugars) is discouraged by nutritionists. Candy bars, cookies and cakes are loaded with sugar that, if not burned up by the body, is stored in the adipose tissue as fat, which is exactly what a dieter wants to avoid.

The difference between simple and complex carbohydrates lies in their molecular makeup. All carbohydrates are compounds of carbon, hydrogen, and oxygen—with hydrogen and oxygen usually appearing in the same ratio as they do in water.

The least complicated of the carbohydrates, the monosaccharides, are also called simple sugars. Fructose, for example, is a monosaccharide and is found naturally in a large number of fruits and in honey. In monosaccharides, the carbohydrate is already so broken down that it is ready for absorption by the body.

Disaccharides, also sugars, are slightly more complex. As the prefix implies, they are actually two monosaccharides bonded together. Before these double sugars (such as sucrose, which is table sugar, and lactose, or milk sugar) can be digested, this bond must be broken. The dissolution of the bond is a quick process, and disaccharides too are rapidly absorbed.

The starches in the carbohydrate family are much more complex. They are made up of thousands of monosaccharides linked together in chains or matrices. Before a potato, for example, can be fully digested, all these linkages must be broken down to free the monosaccharides for use by the body. During digestion, these bonds are cleaved just as rapidly as those in the double sugars (disaccharides), but because of sheer numbers, the entire process is a gradual one. The energy you get from this process is more of a slow, steady burn that the quick burst you get from simple sugars.

The calories obtained from complex carbohydrates (starches) will sustain you over a longer period of time. Partly for that reason, foods containing complex carbohydrates are the preferred fuel for the human engine at best. Besides, they contain many vitamins and minerals and thus have higher nutritional value than snacks like candy or cake. Moreover, many complex carbohydrates also contain fiber, an indigestible plant substance which contains bulk. In addition to the other health benefits, by eating vegetables high in fiber, you'll feel full more quickly.

WEIGHT LOSS SUCCESS #7

Kathy Somerville of Edmonton, Alberta, Canada, battled for four years to lose 20 pounds, though was still not happy with a 25.4 percent of body fat. To lose weight she had to starve herself and knew with some certainty the weight would come back.

So she turned to cycling and before long was riding 2–3 hours a day. Within four months she lost 6.5 percent of body fat and 15 pounds. She reports that the loss improved her mental health "100 percent."

So be sure to eat plenty of starches—potatoes, breads, beans and vegetables—but skip the fatty accompaniments like butter (one pat is 100 calories; one slice of bread is only 60).

Six years ago I attended a lecture for the National Cycling Team given by one of the senior coaches. From the old school, he emphasized eating lots of meat and potatoes before a big race. Based on a survey done at the Coors Classic bicycle race a few years ago, racers seemed to indulge in a lot of carbohydrates as part of their prerace strategy. Some of the favorites include: cereal, fruit and juice (or bread or pancakes and fruit), steak and rice (or chicken and rice), eggs and pancakes (or French toast, oatmeal, etc.), pancakes and waffles, and pastry.

Jacques Boyer and Connie Carpenter, both tops in their field, tend to avoid greasy foods, refined sugars, heavy processing and red meat. Both emphasize whole grains, fresh fruit and vegetables. It hasn't slowed them down.

Caloric Needs. Having heard that the racer who trains three to five hours a day may need 1,500 to 2,000 more calories of energy, less active cyclists often assume that they need more calories than they really do. You'll want to keep careful track of what you're eating and your cycling mileage in your training log to make sure you're not overdoing it at the dinner table.

When the weekend rolls around, you may spend hours in the saddle. Obviously with this increased activity comes an increased energy requirement, and the rider may need to consume more calories to satisfy it. An excellent energy source is the naturally occurring sugars in fruits. And, if you like to indulge in cakes and cookies from time to time, this is the ideal opportunity to get away with it when you can use the extra calories.

Again, if you are concerned about getting needed vitamins and minerals, remember that fresh fruits are rich in nutrients. Figure an orange, which you can easily toss in a bike bag or stick in your jersey pocket, at 65 calories for a medium-sized one, and a banana at 100 calories. Remember too that your body carries stored energy in the form of glycogen, so that if you are merely going to ride a day, you don't have to try to eat as many calories as you burn if you are somewhat higher than your ideal weight. You can experiment to see what sorts of energy foods agree with you when you ride, and just how much you need to eat when riding to avoid lightheadedness and lethargy; don't forget your brain depends on a certain blood sugar level from carbohydrates for proper functioning.

When Monday morning arrives or after the tour is finished, it's back to the normal eating regimen lest you care to add a few extra pounds to carry uphill. Here's why. When you are not actually burning a lot of calories with exercise, that piece of chocolate cake floods your system with a surplus of carbohydrate subunits since it is so quickly digested.

What happens to this surplus fuel? It may be used to replace depleted glycogen stores in the active racer or long-distance rider. But the exertions of a day which is only moderately active cannot be expected to deplete glycogen reserves. In this case, the glycogen stores could already be "full up" and the excess simple sugars will be converted to fat.

In other words, if you are on an exercise program and *gaining* weight, you know you're overdoing it in the nutrition department.

A Few Suggestions. There are a few other hints to help achieve weight loss.

• Read the labels on the food you buy. This can be a real education. Remember that the predominant ingredient is listed first on the package, and the others follow in decreasing order. In far more products than you may expect, sugar will appear in large proportion and in a variety of forms—as sucrose, glucose, maltose, dextrose, lactose, fructose, and syrups, as well as the familiar honey.

Unfortunately, convenience foods often give nutrition a double whammy. Not only are calories added, but important nutrients are taken out. Once you start examining the labels, you may find you need to select convenience foods more carefully and to do more of your own cooking from scratch.

• Reduce dietary fat. The biggest source of calories in your diet is probably high-fat foods. Some of these, such as cookies, cakes, ice cream, and butter, are obvious culprits. But others, such as whole milk, avocados, red meat, and peanut butter, may seem to be too good for us to pass up. No one is saying you should never eat fatty foods, but the truth is that we need little fat to fulfill daily requirements. Our bodies can store almost inexhaustible amounts of fat, so we don't need to eat a great deal to replenish our supply on a daily basis.

• Make sensible food choices. A glass of skim milk has half the calories of whole milk, yet supplies the equivalent nutrients. Mashed potatoes are less fattening than french fries, and passing up the extra pad of butter will save you 100 calories.

You can reduce your total fat intake by eating less animal fat. Trim fat from meat before cooking. Choose among lean meats, fish, poultry, and protein-rich lentils and dried beans rather than red meat and pork. You'll still satisfy your protein requirements, but at half the calories.

It's a good idea to use low-fat and skim milk products whenever possible. Substitute the less-fattening cottage cheese for cream cheese. Drink two-percent skim milk. Eat fewer eggs and less butterfat and other high-cholesterol foods.

• Reduce the size of your portions by choosing the small steak over the large. If you must have pie, take half the size of a normal piece. Skip the concentrated sweets and desserts and cut down on snacks, particularly the chips and pretzels so high in salt and fat content. It's also a good idea to eat four or five small meals rather than three large ones in the course of a day.

In a University of Minnesota study, people fed one 2,000-calorie meal a day in the morning lost weight. When the same people were fed the same meal in the evening in a later study, they lost less or even gained weight. So when you choose to chow-down is important.

• Finally, eat a varied diet. Choosing foods from all the food groups makes not only for nutritious, but interesting meals.

The more we learn about nutrition, it becomes increasingly obvious that personal tastes play a large part in how one eats. "I once knew a rider who lived almost entirely on oranges and wheat germ," recalled coach Norman Shiel. "Nothing that I could say would convince him that his diet was less than perfect or that the food being served at the training camp was not only excellent but had been prepared with the athlete in mind. He lasted a little over three days before having to return home feeling rather poorly. I have always remembered that rider and often wonder if he is still alive."

I am not recommending a diet of oranges and wheat germ. I am suggesting you find the combination of food and calories that suits you. I personally know hundreds of cyclists who, when they are putting in 100-to-150-mile weeks, don't worry a great deal about the amount and number of calories. Sure, they are smart enough and won't neglect the minimum standards of good nutrition. On the other hand, many seem to consume beer and pizza far beyond what the charts indicate as acceptable.

Do these cyclists know something we don't? Probably not. Most are at optimum weight and cycling enough to keep their weight down and BMR up. They know what foods work for them and what don't. I recall before my first running marathon someone recommended that I really indulge heavily in yogurt the week before the race. My reward: 26 miles of gas pains. That was a long time ago.

You know your body. Listen to it. After monitoring your weight loss for a year, you will know what you have to do to keep your weight off. To a certain extent it's a matter of arithmetic. After that, our individual differences come into play. Know thyself.

To be preoccupied with weight loss in the beginning is a very good thing: it gives you a goal. Weight is what you see and feel; it's as real and as palpable as the great outdoors. But, as you lose weight, you also decrease your risk of diabetes, stroke, high blood pressure and hypertension. As you take off pounds, your resting pulse and blood pressure will come down, unless there's an organic problem.

Cycling is not mechanical, providing a one-to-one relationship between an effort and a reward. If you go for a two-hour Sunday ride and burn up 800 calories, you have earned an immediate reward. Beyond that, consider the value of cycling with friends, moving under your own power across real estate you used to cross by car.

In the long run it is these additional benefits that will keep you with the sport long after your dieting friends have embraced another fad. In a fundamental sense cycling provides a psychological support system for weight watchers. While you are waiting for the weight to come off—and it won't be long—you will gain many additional benefits. Cycling will transform you from the inside out. It can make you a new person.

15

That Extra Kick

Within 20 miles of the finish line, John Howard knew he was going to win the 1971 Pan-Am road race. He just wasn't sure how. A Brazilian had broken away from the pack, and was following closely behind. John uncorked his water bottle and swallowed a mixture of coffee and cognac so strong it made fraternity party punch seem like Kool-Aid. He increased his speed, finishing 30 seconds ahead of his competition. He later admitted the race's outcome could have been completely different if he hadn't gulped down some coffee. "I was hyped to the gills on caffeine," he says, "and after the race, I felt depleted, totally." But he had never felt so good about feeling bad. After all, he had won the gold medal.

John Howard wasn't the first—nor will he be the last—to use caffeine to stimulate his cycling performance. In fact, the International Olympic Committee (IOC) removed caffeine from its list of banned substances a few years ago, possibly due to the acceptance and use of coffee, a main source of caffeine, by millions of people around the world.

Evidence shows that even a decade after Howard's gold-medal winning ride cyclists are still experimenting with special diet and drugs to improve their performance. Some, like Howard, may drink a cup or two of coffee before or during a long race for an extra kick.

Others will try "carbo-loading," a dietary regimen that involves exercising to exhaustion and then eating plenty of carbohydrates in an attempt to supersaturate the muscles with precious "high-octane" carbohydrate fuel.

And even at the Olympic Training Center (OTC), sports nutritionist Ann Grandjean said she found a surprising number of high-caliber cyclists who ingested everything from bee pollen to *sand* in an attempt to ride faster with less fatigue.

What's the truth about these substances? Can they really give cyclists a winning edge? Over the year I've asked a panel of experts: Ann Grandjean and Karen Fleischer (Lenox Hill Sports Medicine Clinic); coaches Ed Burke, Clement Kaplan and Tom Dickson, M.D. (Medical Director for the Lehigh County Velodrome in Pennsylvania); and Olympic-caliber riders Brent Emery, Steve Tilford and Roy Knickman.

They concluded that there are no miracles in training, only hard work. Still, whether you're a recreational rider or racer, occasionally adding extra carbohydrates and vitamins to your diet may at some point be beneficial. The trick is to determine the best path to success. You be the judge.

Carbo-Loading. When Peter Van Handel was a student at Ball State University in the early 1970s, he helped David Costill, Ph.D., a muscle physiologist, conduct many experiments with athletes to find a way to improve their performance.

Costill was among the first in this country to look at carbo-loading, an exercise and dietary regimen advanced by Swedish researchers. Athletes followed strict guidelines. On the seventh day before an event, they exercised to exhaustion the muscles used in competition. This emptied them of glycogen, a carbohydrate fuel stored in the muscles and liver. For the next three days, they exercised lightly and ate nothing but fat and protein foods, which don't readily form glycogen (these three days are called the "depletion phase").

The theory was that the muscles, like a sponge, could be wrung dry of all carbohydrate reserves through an exhaustive workout and by eating mostly protein and fat for several days. The athletes then returned to a high-carbohydrate menu in hopes of supersaturating their muscles with carbohydrate substances. You'll recall that carbohydrates in their metabolized form are the preferred fuel in exercise as they require little oxygen to burn.

In a laboratory setting, carbo-loading did indeed work. Athletes rode longer and felt more refreshed during exhaustive workouts on a stationary bike when fueled by a carbo-load regimen. But outside the university, runners and cyclists who put carbo-loading to the test unhappily reported setbacks in their own training.

It was particularly difficult for cyclists to adhere to the depletion part of the program in which they ate primarily protein and fats for three days. Riders accustomed to eating mostly carbohydrates complained that the high-fat foods like meat, milk, cheese and oil sat in their gut and took a long time to digest. Even more serious were tales of cyclists experiencing dizziness and confusion during the depletion phase.

"When you're not eating enough carbohydrates, your blood sugar (glucose) level drops," explained Ed Burke, currently the Sportsmedicine Coordinator for the United States Cycling Federation (USCF), who started out in cycling as a racer in the early seventies:

> Glucose is necessary in keeping the brain and neurological system functioning properly.
>
> It's not surprising that athletes reported feeling

> dizzy and lethargic. Some riders were even passing out during the depletion phase of carbo-loading when they simply weren't eating enough carbohydrates.
>
> I know myself how hard it was to maintain a high protein and fat diet when carbo-loading. I remember going out for a three-hour bike ride and I could barely pedal! I just felt weak and washed out!

The debate about the pros and cons of carbohydrate-loading continued. In the late 1970s, Ball State University researchers tackled the question of carbo-loading once again. This time they recruited six better than average marathon runners, who were subjected to three different trial diets coupled with identical exercise programs. The first trial (A) used the strict loading regimen of three days of a low (15 percent) carbohydrate diet followed by three days of a high (70 percent) carbohydrate diet. The second trial (B) involved a mixed (50 percent) carbohydrate diet for three days followed by a high (70 percent) carbohydrate diet. The third trial (C) involved a mixed (50 percent) diet for six days.

The tests culminated in a 13-mile run on a dirt 220-yard track at the Ball State Field House. Among other things, the researchers saw that in Trial B, the subjects were able to store high levels of carbohydrate fuel (glucose and glycogen) *without* undergoing the arduous depletion part of the carbo-loading regimen. In effect, athletes could substantially increase their carbohydrate stores simply by eating plenty of carbohydrate-rich foods, including pastas and whole-grain breads, three days before an endurance event.

What does this data suggest to the recreational cyclist? Among other things, Costill concluded that *carbo-loading is only useful when you're participating in an event of one and a half to two hours or longer in duration*. In shorter events, diet wasn't really a major factor in performance. If you use your bike solely for commuting or for short recreational rides, stick to a normal diet.

But if you're training for a century (100 miles) or a long tour, a carbo-loading regimen will help you ride longer with less fatigue. However, there are a few steps to carbo-load properly:

Exercise to exhaustion. Four to five days before the tour or century starts, exercise your muscles to exhaustion. There's no strict formula as to how long to bicycle. Peter Van Handel, currently a researcher at the Colorado Springs Sportsmedicine Division, suggests riding several hours "at a real good clip" to burn up carbohydrate fuel stores.

Skip the depletion phase completely. As I've already pointed out, Costill's recent studies showed athletes could increase their muscle glycogen stores and blood glucose levels simply by eating a high-carbohydrate (70 percent) diet for several days following exhaustive exercise. Your carbohydrate intake should be determined by body weight: For each kilogram (2.2 pounds) of body weight, eat 6 or 7 grams of carbohydrates daily until the event. (It's not hard to apply this arithmetic to what's on your table. The labels on most packaged food list grams of carbohydrate per serving. Plus, the U.S. Department of Agriculture has paperback books which list carbohydrate content for all kinds of food.)

Taper off in your training for a few days. If you continue to exercise hard in the few days before the event, you'll use up all the glycogen reserves that you're trying to store! Van Handel advises a period of "relative rest" where you take short spins to keep your form intact but don't deplete the glycogen reserves in the muscles.

Eat a variety of carbohydrates before, during and after the event. You can get the majority of carbohydrate calories by eating fruits and vegetables, pastas and legumes, which not only provide energy but possess the vitamins, minerals and other nutrients necessary for good health.

But don't forget the simple sugars found in candy bars, cookies and other sweets. These so-called "junk foods" provide carbohydrate calories without bulk. "It's thought that there's already too much sugar in the American diet, but a little won't hurt," Van Handel pointed out. "Just don't go overboard."

It's also a good idea to carry along small snacks on the ride, including small sections of oranges and apples, tarts, cookies, granola and the like to replenish glycogen stores while you ride.

Finally, eating carbohydrates is especially important after an endurance event. Even well-conditioned people who have eaten the right things before and during their ride will have depleted the glycogen from their muscles. The way to restore the fuel for more exercise is to emphasize carbohydrates in daily diet. In fact, try to eat 500 to 600 grams of carbohydrate per day for several days following an endurance event. That and lots of rest will help the cyclist recover from even the most grueling event in record time.

Caffeine.   There are some cyclists who attribute a good performance to factors that include, among other things, drinking coffee, a main source of caffeine. For example, a few years ago, racer David Mayer-Oakes told a story of being stranded in Chicago, with only $45 in his pocket and two days to go before a 40-mile criterium. He woke up sleeping on the floor of a friend's hotel room, scheming to win the race's $1,000 purse. Without that money, his only mode of transportation home would be his thumb. He filled his water bottle with strong coffee before the race and claims caffeine engineered his victory. "I knew I had to win, and coffee would carry me all the way to the top, and it did," he says.

The casual cyclist might be surprised to hear such wonders ascribed to caffeine. But, according to Ed Burke, caffeine has been a stimulant for racers for years. "I don't want to say that racers need it, but some take it for that extra kick in the last laps."

Indeed, a survey conducted by *Bicycling* magazine showed 37 percent of those racers who rode in the Coors Classic favored some type of caffeinated beverage (tea, tea with honey, cola, coffee) during races for extra punch. Seven of the 34 racers who indicated this preference said it was during the last stages, or only in long races, that they used caffeine.

Nonetheless, although a rider like Mayer-Oakes claims caffeine helps his performance, he's not exactly sure why. That's not surprising. For years scientists weren't certain either. They knew caffeine, like amphetamine, was a drug which stimulates the central nervous system and contracts the heart muscle at a quicker pace. More recently, researchers like David Costill began to look at the influence of caffeine on fat metabolism. Although he was not the first to make the connection between caffeine and quick energy, his were among the first laboratory tests to clearly show caffeine improved athletic performance. In fact, using trained cyclists on bicycle ergometers, Costell found those who ingested caffeine improved their total exercise time by 19 percent.

In effect, he showed that caffeine, under the right conditions, could help burn a greater percentage of body fat in the form of free fatty acids. Although the active cyclist burns a mixture of both carbohydrates (glycogen) and fats (free fatty acids) in exercise, free fatty acids require a great deal of oxygen to "combust." (Since carbohydrate requires little oxygen, it is a preferred fuel in exercise.)

Unfortunately, our body stores only limited amounts of carbohydrate fuel but an inexhaustible supply of fat. The discovery that caffeine helped "tap" these fat stores for the cyclist was hailed as a milestone in exercise physiology.

But it was discovered there were several drawbacks to using caffeine too. First, caffeine is a diuretic, meaning it helps urine pass through the kidneys quickly and encourages dehydration. In longer races, frequent rest stops are an annoyance. Moreover, the cyclist will have to keep careful tabs on his intake of water, making sure he isn't losing fluids too quickly because of the caffeine's diuretic effects.

Moreover, drinking coffee on an empty stomach can sometimes provoke intestinal cramps, as David Mayer-Oakes can attest. "On mornings when I only drink coffee and take long rides," he says, "my stomach might feel upset. It usually passes."

In some instances, caffeine can actually do more harm than good. "Some people who are hypersensitive to caffeine will actually perform worse under the influence of coffee," says William Fink, a researcher at Ball State who works with Costill. "When taken in the right amount (estimated to be approximately two cups of coffee), the caffeine will enhance the release of fatty acids and spares muscle glycogen. An overdose, however, becomes a stress of its own, where the body responds by drawing on the muscle glycogen more rapidly. Athletes have to go on their own experience with the drug to gauge whether it will work for them."

So Fink emphasizes that the effects of caffeine vary with the individual, and that there is no way to predict accurately the scope of caffeine's benefits. Short of using radioactive tracers, physiologists still can't determine how great an influx of fatty acids is present after ingesting caffeine. Fink suggested caffeine's effects on the release of fatty acids "isn't as drastic as some people like to think."

Ed Burke advises most cyclists to ignore the caffeine craze as a method to improve performance. "While you're touring, you won't need coffee at all," he suggests, "because you're working at a steady, leisurely pace, which will help burn fats away.

"The only time I encourage a racer to ingest caffeine is in a stage race, for example, with a national team, when the rider may be in his seventh day and having a hard time getting his energy up for the last laps."

As a matter of fact, researchers suggest the best way to tap the unlimited fat stores in your body is by training. Take plenty of long rides at a moderate pace and you'll use up blood sugars and muscle glycogen and teach your body to rely on fatty acids.

"The trained individual finds activities effortless at speeds where the untrained jogger or cyclist experiences breathlessness and fatigue," points out Daniel J. Hanley, M.D., a resident in neurology at Johns Hopkins. Gradually, what was maximum effort for a cyclist will become less strenuous, as his body learns to commandeer oxygen more rapidly. Researchers aren't quite sure how this happens biologically, although one thing we know is that with training, the cyclist actually increases the number of capillary blood vessels which carry oxygen and fatty acids to the muscles. With a greater circulation of oxygen, fats can be burned more rapidly.

At Costill's laboratory, muscle physiologists have also observed that the trained muscle will begin to adapt itself for burning fats. "We've noticed that with training, the muscle cell itself will actually store more fat to be burned," said one assistant. With conditioning the cyclist can also increase the number of the muscle cell mitochondria, tiny subcellular structures which burn fatty acids inside the muscle.

All these factors can influence an athlete's fat-burning capacity. It's estimated that a cyclist with limited training will probably burn approximately 45 percent fats, 45 percent carbohydrates and 10 percent protein on long, easy rides. But by weeks of conditioning through long, steady rides the body gradually adjusts until it's burning about 60 percent fats, 30 percent carbohydrates, and 10 percent protein.

The moral? Caffeine may work wonders for *you*, but it's no substitute for regular training.

Extra Vitamins.   There are many other substances available to the cyclist to improve performance. Some, like anabolic steroids, have been banned internationally. Others, like ephedrine, are available over the counter in either oral or spray form. (Ephedrine stimulates the release of adrenaline and is thought to enhance energy, although that remains unproven.)

For the recreational cyclist, these substances are exotic and it is unlikely they'll creep into your training program. It is far more plausible that you—like many riders—will invest in vitamin supplements to give you vigor.

But do you really need them? Physicians and nutritionists are frequently at odds about what type and in what dosages vitamins are necessary for an athletic person. One panel of experts suggests that before taking supplements, a recreational cyclist's first step should be to eat a balanced diet. It helps to eat a variety of foods too. Recent studies indicate that eating a vitamin-rich food does not always mean your body will make full use of its benefits.

"I'd say American cyclists have a pretty clear idea what vitamins can and can't do for them," says Ed Burke. "European cyclists, on the other hand, are still using so many far-fetched approaches. Why, they're even putting vitamins in their water bottles!"

Nonetheless, while Burke was quick to point out vitamin supplements aren't necessary to drink during the race itself, he did say active cyclists may want to take a multivitamin plus iron every day as good insurance.

"The vitamin question is a very complex problem," he explained.

> You're looking at highly individual circumstances, such as how the cyclist eats, his own enzyme systems, his vitamin, fluid, and food levels, and how he feels to determine whether he needs vitamins and in what amount. That's why we suggest that a multivitamin tablet doesn't hurt.
>
> [Massive amounts] of supplements are another thing altogether. Some cyclists take extra vitamins B and C because they're training hard and may not have time to eat properly. But don't go overboard.

"We don't really start to worry unless we see a cyclist taking ten times the RDA (Recommended Daily Allowance) in certain vitamins and minerals," nutritionist Ann Grandjean, who's spent the past year working with Olympic cyclists, explains.

> Ten times is the cutoff point for what we call the "therapeutic value" of supplements. Doses that exceed this amount probably are not helping the cyclist at all.
>
> If a cyclist is taking massive doses of a supplement, we'll recommend blood tests to determine to what degree the cyclist is storing or excreting that particular vitamin or mineral.
>
> We're especially concerned when they're taking large doses of the fat-soluble vitamins A, D, E and K, which are transported by fat and stored in several sites in the body, including the liver and adipose tissue. We think water-soluble vitamins (B and C) are less dangerous because excesses are excreted in the urine, but there's still ongoing laboratory research in this area.

Grandjean's work with the cyclists then is twofold: to discourage cyclists from overloading on vitamin and mineral supplements and at the same time come up with a balanced nutritious diet they can train on and live with.

It's not always easy. "I once saw an athlete who took *117* times the recommended dose of certain vitamins. It's hard to convince them that vitamins in that dosage won't give them a winning edge." Of particular interest to Grandjean are the substances which have little or no nutritional value whatever, such as seaweed and bee pollen. "In fact, I saw a cyclist who was taking silica tablets which were supposed to 'aid digestion and improve performance.' Silica is sand!

"Providing it's not *dangerous*, I usually feel it's the cyclist's business. There's a psychological side to nutrition, where a cyclist sometimes eats something thinking it will help him ride better, and perhaps it does."

16

Indoors and Out: Your Total Fitness Program

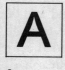

A pproximately 60 million Americans consider themselves recreational cyclists, meaning they cycle a few times a year. That practice might bring them pleasure, but it won't bring them fitness.

For most Americans the run of the seasons is a joy. At the same time, late fall and winter can significantly curtail your outside cycling program. A few years ago that might have been a problem but today, with the availability of so many sophisticated indoor exercise guides, as well as a second generation of exercise bikes, cycling all year is a possibility and a pleasure.

On the other hand, you might want cycling at the core of your exercise program and, during the year or during the off-season, balance your cycling with running, cross-country skiing or other compatible sports. In this chapter I will discuss all these options.

I should say that you can cycle outdoors most months of the year in most climates. Cycling offers an array of cool weather gear that will make riding in the fall and winter a pleasant experience.

But if you do move indoors in October or November, you have many options. You can hook up your road bike to a wind-load simulator such as discussed in the chapter on measuring your fitness. You could ride bicycle rollers. Or you could buy an exercise bike. Obviously, you could make use of the exercise bikes at your local YMCA or health club. These institutions usually have Monarch or other ergometers which enable you to get a good workout. On the other hand, I've found that parking my Monarch in front of the television keeps me honest in the winter. If I want to watch a football game, I have to exercise. To be sure, a Monarch can cost over $700, but I consider it a lifetime investment in health for my family.

Some cyclists want to take a little time off the bike in the winter. Most racers do this for physical and psychological reasons. A professional racer might have cycled 20,000 miles during the course of a season and needs time to recuperate. You might want a change of pace and there's nothing wrong with that. Quite likely, due to your schedule or circumstance, you probably have engaged in compatible activities throughout the year, particularly when you have been unable to get on the bike.

COMPATIBLE SPORTS

Running. I know many cyclists who use running as a complementary activity. I'm one of them. I ride as often as I can, but when I travel, I take along my running shoes. I usually run at least one marathon a year and a number of shorter races. I find running nicely complements my cycling. In fact, many of the editors on the *Bicycling* magazine staff run for the same reasons.

If you get off your bike in the fall and jump into your running shoes, expecting to enjoy the same kind of rhythm and cadence, you're probably in for a surprise. It will take you a few weeks to adjust to a running schedule, unless you have run a bit during the rest of the year. As Canadian racer Hugh Walton points out, "Your heart's in shape, everything's in shape except the little muscles in your legs. They hurt like crazy."

The fact is, your lower body takes a pounding when running that it is not used to from cycling, and it will take some time for you to adjust. John Howard, veteran racing champion and Ironman Triathlon winner, ran successfully in high school but didn't get back to the sport until he trained for the Hawaii Ironman contest. He acknowledged that he started with a lot of enthusiasm. "I tried to do too much and ended up with shin splints."

Howard recommends a more gradual approach, beginning the first day running a quarter of a mile and increasing your distance to a half-mile by the end of the week. Then to a mile and so on. Other authorities suggest a run-walk or a slow run schedule for the first few weeks.

In your transition from cycling to running it is important that you stretch a great deal; remember that cycling involves primarily the front muscles in your legs while running, the hamstrings and the calves. In a survey taken of cyclists-runners, the majority said that they stretched before and after running, while a few said they stretched before cycling.

I'll discuss stretching in some detail a little later but in your transition from cycling to running, do a couple of basic stretches. Lean against a wall and inch backward until you feel your calves stretch. Hold that position for a few seconds. Another useful stretch is the leg extension where you put a foot up on a chair, table or step and bring your trunk down gently.

If you are getting back into running after a long layoff or are just beginning, go easy at first. Your body's in shape but your legs must adjust. Try the walk-run routine for a couple of weeks. If you don't push yourself, you can increase your mileage quickly. Within a month you should be running at your pace at least 3–4 times a week for forty-minute sessions. That will help you maintain your level of cardiovascular conditioning. If you've been at all competitive in cycling, you will likely be drawn to running races, particularly the 10k. Once your legs are accustomed to the pace, participate in some of these races. They will help keep you honest and are a fine diversion.

Depending on your schedule you might want to use running throughout the year to supplement your cycling and general fitness. While there is no substitute for time in the saddle, a modest running program during the season will benefit your cycling, particularly on the hills. Cycling builds up the quadriceps—the muscles in front of the thighs. In fact, almost all the training defects of running will transfer to cycling. To maintain my running legs I run two to three times a week year-round, even when I'm cycling 150 miles a week. I find I'm much stronger because of this dual training. I would recommend a similar program for you, unless you cannot run due to musculoskeletal imbalance.

Cross-country Skiing.   Many cycling enthusiasts run in the off-season but many more participate in cross-country skiing. The same leg muscles that propel you on a bike propel the cross-country skier. An added benefit is that your shoulder and arm muscles also get a good workout.

Though a lot of cyclists participate in cross-country skiing, the transition is not quite as easy as to running. Equipment could be a problem, but that is not the province of this book. I suggest you consult *Cross-Country Ski Gear* by Michael Brady, available in most libraries.

Even if you have the right equipment, you won't be able to simply jump off your bike and onto skis. John Lloyd, a cross-country ski instructor, suggests you get ready for the sport by doing a lot of brisk walking, 20 to 30 minutes, five days a week. At the same time keep your hands free so you can swing your arms to simulate the poling motions. Your left arm swings forward with the right leg and vice versa.

After a couple of weeks you will be ready for a gentle

jogging program, slow enough to carry on a conversation. Start at 20-minute sessions and work up to 45 minutes. As with brisk walking, you have to be attentive to your upper body coordination. In anticipation of skiing, you have to simulate the same arm movements, which will take some practice because that's not how most of us run. When you are comfortable with your jogging, try to move up a little on your toes. Lloyd suggests you "thrust yourself off the ball of your foot, curling your toes under as if running barefoot on the beach. This simulates the motion of skiing."

At this point you can add ski poles to your jogging and run on a soft surface so you can plant your poles. With proper preparation you can earn very high cardiovascular benefits from cross-country skiing.

INDOOR OPTIONS

No matter what the inducements of other activities, cyclists will insist on riding indoors. For years a popular training device has been bicycle rollers, which consist of cylindrical drums in a frame. The bike rests on the drums and drives them through a pulley system.

Rollers are popular all over the world. At the training camp for professional cyclists in Japan a large barnlike building houses dozens of sets of rollers for use when it is raining. As the director of the training camp told me, the racers don't use the rollers to increase their cardiovascular performance; they use them for cadence and some conditioning.

Len Vreeland, who holds the Master's record for riding on the rollers 717 miles in 24 hours at age 46, recommends roller riding as a way to keep your high rpm, fluid pedaling motion during the off-season, particularly if you run. "I find with roller riding I am able to maintain my form throughout the winter." Vreeland, a marathon cyclist who crossed the country in 14 days on a recumbent when he was fifty, recommends a warm-up period of five minutes at 90 rpm. Then he picks up the pace to 100 rpm and 120, where he does some wind sprints. As with any form of cycling, vary the program to your needs.

Rollers prove problematic for some people as it's like learning to ride a bike all over again. Because you're actually cycling on rolling drums, this activity requires a great deal of balance. The tendency is to oversteer, a habit that can be corrected in a couple of sessions.

Some people set the rollers up in doorways or close to an object that serves as a safety net. Do whatever is comfortable for you. Think back to an earlier chapter on relaxing on your bike. This holds equally true of roller riding, where a light touch and smooth cadence are essential. For those reasons alone it's good for every serious cyclist to know how to ride rollers.

Like everything else, rollers cost money, about $130. After you have considered all the alternatives for indoor fitness, you will have to decide how to best spend your money. Clearly a device you are not going to use often is not worth the investment. And before you purchase anything, check it out. Many clubs and most bike shops will have rollers for you to try. Take advantage of these opportunities.

At one time roller riding was the only real cycling alternative for the enthusiast. As recently as five years ago the marketplace offered very little in the way of stands or devices that could enable you to use your bike indoors. However, in the last couple of years, these stands, more correctly known as wind-load simulators, permit you to use your own bike. These devices have a common feature: A pair of rotating fans apply resistance to the rear wheel which increases as you increase your speed. Since you have the benefit of using your bicycle gearing, you are working against a resistance that you control. Though your position is fixed in place as you are locked into the stand, you can come close to simulating road riding conditions without the hills. Thus, these training devices offer significant fitness advantages over rollers.

Physiologist Ed Burke employed six racers to test whether rollers or Racer Mate, a wind-load simulator, was better. Six racers were tested at the Work Physiology Laboratory, Ohio State University, to determine whether rollers or wind-load simulator (Racer Mate) created a desired training effect. On the rollers the racers' mean heart rate was 70 percent and 76 percent while pedaling in a 52-17, 52-15, and 52-13 gear ratio. On the Racer Mate heart rates were measured at 72 percent, 84 percent and 97 percent at the same workload. Oxygen consumption was significantly higher when cyclists used the Racer Mate.

Thus, while rollers put some demonstrable stress on the cardiovascular system, a Racer Mate will give you a better workout.

The Racer Mate is just one of a number of brands currently available. Others include: the Turbo Trainer, the Road Simulator, the Vetta Trainer and the J.C.I. X-Air Stand. Prices vary considerably, depending on whether you buy the full system with options. You can purchase the Racer Mate and wind-load device for about $150, which is a good bargain. In fact, since these devices won't have to take the abuse that comes with outside use, they should have a very long life. There is a Turbo Trainer in the Fitness Center where I work and it has been ridden by hundreds of riders many thousands of miles, showing few signs of wear.

I should add that a second generation of rollers is being introduced, ones that offer the benefits of roller riding with some resistance. Among these are the Tac rollers and the Kreitler Headwind system. You can inspect many of these units at your retail bike shop. I've listed manufacturers' addresses in the Appendix for your convenience.

Whatever system you use, the wind-load simulators have made it possible to get a good workout indoors, while riding a bike you are familiar with. In the past people have been reluctant to use indoor training devices because there was no reliable way to measure fitness. That excuse is no longer relevant. Neither is boredom. You can do just about anything on these indoor units you can do on your road bike.

A key to successful indoor training is to establish a routine and schedule for yourself. What follows is a sample one-hour indoor workout suggested by endurance cyclist and author Rob Templin and Hannah North, racer. Nothing is written in stone. If you are starting your indoor fitness program after a full season on the road, this schedule should post few difficulties. However, if you are starting indoors, all the recommendations offered in the earlier chapter apply, including a medical checkup if appropriate.

SAMPLE WORKOUT

1. *10–15 Minutes:* A proper warm-up, an obvious necessity whether inside or out on the road, should begin any workout. Slowly increase the gears but always in a cadence close to 90–100 rpm. To determine cadence, several of the electronic devices come in handy. Since most wind-simulator stands require removal of the front wheel, you'll have to mount the speed sensor that most computers use there on the rear wheel if you want the speed function. The computers help to reduce the problem of wandering minds, making riding a little more fun. If you don't want the expense of installing a computer, the old standby of using a clock to count pedal strokes will do.

2. *15 Minutes:* Time trial at a steady pace without going into oxygen debt. Try to maintain the same cadence as previously, but using the biggest gears possible.

3. *10 Minutes:* Intervals are next. Hannah North recommends eight of them: 30 seconds at maximum effort, followed by one minute of easy spinning for recovery, etc.

4. *5–10 Minutes:* Recovery time—proceed as in warm-up.

5. *5–10 Minutes:* Specialty training. You can make this the "fun" time to work on whatever you want—sprints, jumps, "ghost tag" (chasing an imaginary rider), etc.

6. *10 Minutes:* Cool-down time. Get right off the bike afterward and dry off or shower.

How you deal with indoor training depends to a great extent on your imagination. If it helps you to listen to music, watch television, or read, take your pick. Just don't become so engrossed in the diversion that you neglect your mission.

The preceding workout is exactly that; it is meant to make you work. Of course, you probably wouldn't want to follow that kind of routine every day. As on the road, one day you might want to try some Long Steady Distance. Whatever approach you take, remember you'll have to exercise at least three or four times a week for an hour or thereabouts if you want to maintain (or reach) your fitness level.

If you are really ambitious you might consider the indoor workout undertaken by Lon Halderman, one of the premier ultramarathon cyclists in the world. He followed this routine while training for his victory in the Great

American Bicycle Race in 1983. Halderman used a Road Machine, though you could use a Racer Mate, a Turbo Trainer or rollers with high resistance. The latter can't be used for the standing parts of the routine. You should know that Halderman commutes 42 miles to work and takes the long way home, churning up the last 10 miles in a whopping 108 gear.

Miles	RPM	Gear	
0-1	80-90	70-80	Warm-up in a gear you can spin in proportion to your body weight. Hands on top of bars.
1-2	90-100	70-80	Spin a little faster with your hands still on top of bars.
2-3	90-100	70-80	Ride with your hands on the drops and your forearms parallel to the floor. This position helps develop the tricep strength to support your body and the lower back flexibility needed to hold a streamlined position at a high rpm.
3-3½	80	90-100	In a higher gear, now stand up and pretend you are riding a unicycle. Your hands can rest on the wall next to you only for balance. Hold this speed for a half mile if possible, and don't bob or sway from side to side but keep your head steady.
3½-4	80	90-100	Recover sitting down and spin smoothly for a half mile.

Miles	RPM	Gear	
4-4½	100	90-100	Increase your speed and rpm.
4½-5	120	90-100	Sprint and hold for as long as possible, half a mile.
5-5½	100	80-90	Recover while spinning. Hands on drops.
5½-6	80	80-90	Left leg only, half a mile.
6-6½	80	80-90	Right leg only, half a mile.
6½-7	90	80-90	Steady prepare for sprint.
7-7½	120	90-100	Sprint for half a mile.
7½-8	100	80-90	Steady half a mile.
8-8½	80	90-100	Standing again, half a mile.
8½-9	100	90-100	Steady half a mile.
9-9½	120	90-100	Last bit sprint, half a mile.
9½-10	80	80-90	Warm-down, easy pedaling.

As I noted before, more and more clubs are purchasing Racer Mates or similar devices for serious training. The Dick Lane Velodrome in Atlanta, Georgia, purchased a number of Racer Mates for use by track riders, who rode in a room with a big 60-second clock that helped them keep in the mood. For example, a rider would do a set interval and then take his pulse, which was easy because of the large clock.

Among other things, the racers played games, such as

matching each other's pedal strokes—anything to keep from getting bored. If the rider's specialty was the 4,000-meter event, he had to show improvement in his time.

While you might not be getting ready for the Olympics, there is no reason you cannot vary your schedule or type of riding to suit your mood. Keep your indoor riding interesting and playful. You can still get a great workout but there's no reason to be glum.

A word of caution: Though 25 mph on a Racer Mate is not the same as 25 mph on the road, it is still pretty fast. You can work hard on a wind-load training device without really knowing it. For that reason, some coaches actually suggest using both the device and rollers on alternate days. That might be good advice for the competitive riders, but not for the recreational cyclist. If you are using a training device and particularly if you are riding every day, you should follow the same hard and easy routine discussed in an earlier chapter. Some days you might simply want to put in time in the saddle, reading a book, without too much attention to your THR. Other days you might want to mix in some intervals. If you have a cadence meter or a metronome, this would be a good time to use it. You might play a little. Imagine you're participating in a fast ride for 20 to 30 minutes. Orchestrate your pedal cadence. Change your number of rpms as you might in an actual fast-paced race. Try to jump and break away from the other riders. Sprint to the finish line. (You lost; do it again.)

In a previous chapter I described some of the electronic heart monitors currently available. Depending on the unit you have, indoor cycling is a perfect opportunity to try a pulse monitor because there are none of the weather and motion problems associated with outside use. Being able to check your heart rate and having a monitor with a built-in program of interval training based on your THR could make your indoor cycling performance- and goal-oriented, which is the core of any long-term fitness program.

If for some reason rollers and Racer Mates don't interest you, why not try a third alternative for indoor training: a stationary bicycle. Four or five years ago I probably would not be offering this advice because there were few quality machines on the market. With those available you couldn't really get a vigorous workout. Fortunately, all that has changed. The current crop of stationary bikes are made to order for the fitness-minded.

Receiving a stationary bike for Christmas used to be a gag gift, like that tie you never wore. I heard Howard Cosell say during the broadcast of the Pittsburgh Steelers/ New Orleans Saints game that the Saints quarterback Kenny Stabler was given a stationary bike during the off-season as a joke. Some joke; Stabler opened the 1984 season lighter and in better shape than he enjoyed in years. Chalk one up for the bike.

At *Bicycling* magazine we tested ten stationary bikes ranging from $159 to $2,300. I don't have the space to offer you a full consumer report on the bikes but would be happy to send you a copy if you write to the address listed in the Appendix.

You can imagine with a $2,000 price spread there were some significant differences among the bikes. Given the price, some bikes are probably best suited for health clubs and YMCAs. Most people would probably blink at paying $700 for a Monarch Ergometer, though it's a sturdy bike that would last a lifetime.

The Ergo Metronic 35 at $2,000 might make you blink twice. This machine keeps a computerized record of your rpm, time, mileage and heart rate. The machine responds to your target heart rate and makes the pedaling either easier or more difficult. Big Brother indeed watches you.

In the middle of the spectrum are bikes such as the Air-Dyne from Schwinn, on which the handlebars serve as levers to give your upper body a workout. I know a number of people who use the Air-Dyne and they report good performance. Some use it all year round.

Electronic options are available on some of the reasonably priced bikes. The Pulse Data by Huffy has sensors in the hand grips that give a constant digital reading of your pulse. As you increase your work, you actually watch your heart rate climb.

One advantage of an exercise bike is that more than one person can use it. My wife and I both use the same stationary bike; all we have to do is adjust the seat. A wind-load system would cost you less, but you might not want to secure your bike to the frame—and therefore immobilize it.

Space limitations could be a consideration. Generally speaking, the stationary bike takes up less room than the wind-load device. There are some stationary bikes that actually fold up to be placed in a closet when you are finished. Whatever your choice, it is a buyer's market with a lot of good buys and good choices.

I know some riders who won't use a stationary bike because it doesn't feel like the real thing. I know others who purchase one and then equip it with a familiar saddle and toe clips. To a certain extent, your choice should be dictated by what you want to spend and how much you intend to use it, though keep in mind you won't use an uncomfortable product. I recommend that you don't purchase a bike that flexes too much in the frame. As on the road, that will drain your energy.

One advantage of being in the saddle over the winter is that you won't have to get used to the thing all over again in the spring. That is doubly true if you put your own saddle on the exercise bike. Another advantage is that, if you skip a month or two of exercise, you are back where you started. You lose the beneficial effects very quickly. According to William Fink, Ph.D., of Ball State University's Human Performance Laboratory, "Your resting heart rate will start to climb, the capillaries which opened through exercise will close, and the muscle tissue surrounding the lungs will decrease its capacity to transport oxygen."

Very few people maintain the same intensity of training and conditioning all year round. That is not likely to happen to you if you have a fairly set program and goal. You might decide that your goal over the winter is to maintain your weight and general conditioning. If you are on a *maintenance* program, you might want to mix your activities. You could cycle indoors (or outside) two or three days a week and supplement that with two days of running three to five miles. You might want to add a couple of days of weight work. The most important thing is your objective. If you are content with the maintenance program, that's fine. You have a wide variety of cardiovascular activities to choose from. If, on the other hand, you want to maintain your level of cycling and get ready for some long rides early in the season, then your cycling program should reflect that goal.

If you are using an exercise bike, you should follow the same principles outlined elsewhere. As you would not start out in a high gear, you would not begin your ride against the highest resistance. Choose a resistance level that will let you pedal at 80 to 90 rpm. Get in your base miles, then consider doing sets of intervals.

I usually ride at least two or three times a week on my Monarch during the winter. At least once a week I will do intervals, with no set pattern. I'll usually warm up for about ten kilometers at a low or moderate setting, then I'll increase the resistance and my cadence for set periods of time. Depending on the level of exertion, I might do a minute or two at high resistance and high cadence, and slow down for a minute, then pick up the pace again. I'll do as many sets as my mood dictates, usually eight to ten, followed by a warm-down.

There are any number of variations you can apply to your own program. If you are feeling very good and want a power workout, set the bike on a high resistance and pedal for two to three minutes, slow down and repeat up to six times. You can extend this by doing "jump" training, referring to a racer's act of breaking away from the pack. Set the resistance at maximum and from a full stop pedal to maximum speed and hold for a few seconds. Rest a couple of minutes and repeat, up to ten during a workout.

Consider all these suggestions relative to your constitution. If you are not in fairly good shape you should conduct fewer repetitions at considerably less resistance. You will have to determine that.

You should also consider the physiological consequences of some of these exercises. The specialized training outlined here will in time show up in muscular development of your quadriceps. You might not want this. Many women, including my wife, cycle on stationary bikes for considerable distances at a relatively high rpm and low resistance. My wife is quite conscious of this and is happy to work aerobically on her endurance level. She does not want to do any specialized training because she doesn't want to build up the front of her legs. Long, steady cycling will definitely tone up the legs and buttocks, reaching areas on the inner thigh that running doesn't seem to reach. Therefore, the fact that a certain exercise regimen produces favorable fitness effects (e.g. lower resting pulse) doesn't necessarily mean it is for you. Importantly, you have to decide what you want cycling (or any exercise) to do for you.

FIXED-GEAR TRAINING

Another option for off-season training is to use a fixed-gear bicycle. Unlike your multispeed freewheel bicycle on which the pedals turn only when you turn them, a fixed gear is a direct drive bicycle; when the rear wheel turns, so do the pedals.

On the face of it this kind of bike might seem unnecessary, if not dangerous, though you should know that most European professionals ride up to 1,000 miles in fixed-gear training. The reason for this is that this setup forces you to pedal constantly and smoothly. With one gear available—in the middle range—you are not so likely to get out of the saddle and fight your way up hills. You will feel if the cranks are pulling your feet around and should adjust accordingly. With fixed-gear riding you will be able to concentrate more on pulling up on the pedals, engaging the hamstrings which are important in high rpm cycling.

Fixed-gear cycling will improve your cadence and spin. Since you only have one gear available, you will concentrate on your pedaling, not the gearing. Obviously, you have to choose the terrain carefully.

Fixed-gear training is not for everyone and should not be taken lightly. If you are interested you could get your bike shop mechanic to convert your bike to a fixed gear. You could buy a track—fixed-gear—bike, though you probably would not want to do that unless you intend to engage in track riding.

As with any other form of off- or early-season training, your rides in a fixed gear should be short to moderate. If you are able to get out, take 10-to-20-mile rides. You will find this kind of specialized training very beneficial once you get back on your multispeed bicycle.

WEIGHT AND CIRCUIT PROGRAM

The winter is a good opportunity to take stock of your overall fitness and work on particular muscle groups that need developing and on your flexibility. It would be advisable for all cyclists to include a little flexibility and strength training as a way to stay in shape and to get ready for the next season.

Weight work, particularly on progressive resistance machines such as Universal or Nautilus, has been shown to improve aerobic capacity as well as strength. Researchers have demonstrated that high-resistance, low-repetition weight training has little effect on cardiorespiratory fitness. However, circuit weight training (CWT), which emphasizes low resistance and high repetition, has been shown to improve cardiorespiratory capacity by as much as 17 percent. Similarly, lean body mass increased and fat decreased. Investigators concluded that CWT is a good way to help maintain aerobic fitness (*The Physician and Sportsmedicine*, January, 1981).

Before I outline a modest weight program, a few words about warm-up and cool-down. By and large I have paid little attention to these phases because, done properly, you can warm up and cool down very nicely on a bike. Nonetheless, stretching can be as helpful to a cyclist as a runner and you will find some detailed stretching exercises in the next couple of pages.

What follows is a detailed circuit training program for aerobic and muscular development by Budd Coates, Fitness Director for Rodale Press, Inc. He not only oversees the program, he runs a marathon in 2.14.

The circuit program implies some use of progressive resistance weight common at gyms, YMCAs, and health clubs. The program itself consists of 10 to 12 activity stations performed in a certain order with 35 seconds of aerobic exercise between each station. The purpose of the activity stations is to increase the muscular strength and endurance of your upper, middle and lower body.

To determine what weight you should be working with, you have a couple of options. If you've been cycling all year or engaged in any strenuous aerobic activity, calculate 60 percent of your maximum effort. If you are a beginner, choose a weight that you can use eight times with your upper body and twelve times with your lower body.

You should determine your Target Heart Rate (see again p. 73) before beginning such a program.

TIPS FOR A SUCCESSFUL CIRCUIT PROGRAM

1. Always perform a warm-up and cool-down.
2. Begin the program with one complete cycle only.
3. Perform the Circuit Program three times each week with at least one day of rest between circuits.
4. Each week increase your Circuit Program by one third of the total number of stations.
   Example:
   If your circuit program contains 12 stations, add four the second week for a total of 16, add four more the third week for a total of 20 and four more the fourth week so that you're doing two complete cycles.

5. When you reach 3 complete cycles you should not add any more.
6. Take a six-second pulse at the midpoint and end of each cycle, and after the last station is completed.
7. When you are able to do between 18 and 20 repetitions at any of the lifting stations and you are completing at least two cycles, you should increase the resistance of those stations.

8. Remember to keep a 3–2 ratio between the leg extension and leg curl machines.

Example:

Leg Extension	Leg Curl
2	1
3	2
4	3
5	3
6	4

9. When starting, it is a good idea to perform the same aerobic exercise between each of the stations. When you complete more than two cycles and you maintain your Target Heart Rate, you may alternate between two, three or more aerobic activities.

10. Don't be alarmed if you experience some stiffness the morning after your Circuit Program. This is common, and with time and perseverance it will pass.

WARM-UP

• Relaxation

Lie on back with knees bent.

1. Slowly inhale, hold for two to three seconds and then exhale.
2. Slowly roll head to the left and hold for two to three seconds then roll to the right and hold for two to three seconds. Repeat two more times.
3. Slowly inhale and raise your shoulders toward your ears, hold for two to three seconds and exhale while releasing the shoulders.
4. Repeat step two.
5. Slowly inhale and clench your hands (make a fist)

as tight as possible, hold two to three seconds and exhale while releasing the hands.

6. Repeat step two.

• Stretching

Lie on back with knees bent.

1. Hamstring stretch, single leg.
   a. Bring one knee to your chest, make sure your hips are resting on the floor (no weight on lower foot).
   b. Slowly extend your leg upward until the knee is straight.
   c. Hold for eight to ten seconds.
   d. While straight, lower your leg to the floor and return it to bent knee position.
   e. Repeat with other leg.
   (Perform with bottom leg straight during cool-down)

2. Hamstring and lower back stretch, both legs.
   a. Bring both knees to your chest.
   b. Grasp knees with both hands and pull toward chest.
   c. Hold for eight to ten seconds and release.
   d. Extend both legs upward until knees are straight.
   e. Reach up and grasp both legs, pull toward shoulders but do not allow your knees to bend.
   f. Hold for eight to ten seconds.
   g. While keeping both legs straight slowly lower your legs (should take about eight seconds).

3. Windmills.
   a. With your arms reaching out to the sides lean to left. Put left hand as close to the floor as possible and right hand up. Then return and lean to the right.
   b. Repeat eight to ten times.

4. Trunk twists.
   a. With your arms reaching out to the sides turn to the left as far as possible and look behind, return and turn to the right.
   b. Repeat eight to ten times.

Walk in a large circle.

5. Chest and upper back stretch.
   a. Cross your arms in front of your chest.
   b. Move elbows back behind your chest and double pump.
   c. Open your arms and repeat eight to ten times.

6. Shoulder stretch.
   a. Large arm circles.
      eight to ten forward
      eight to ten backward
   b. Alternate arm circles.
      eight to ten forward
      eight to ten backward

7. Shake arms and legs out and begin the circuit.

COOL-DOWN

1. Get some water if you want and then walk in a large circle.

2. Shake arms and legs out.

3. Shoulder stretch.
   a. Large arm circles.
      eight to ten forward
      eight to ten backward

  b. Alternate arm circles.
      eight to ten forward
      eight to ten backward

4. Chest and upper back stretch.
   a. Cross your arms in front of your chest.
   b. Move elbows back behind your chest and double pump.
   c. Open your arms and repeat eight to ten times.

Standing in a circle.

5. Slowly circle hips to the left (30 seconds).

6. Slowly circle hips to the right (30 seconds).

7. Hip stretch.
   a. Slowly lean to the left as far as possible, feet slightly more than shoulder-width apart.
   b. Hold for eight to ten seconds and return to standing position.
   c. Repeat steps three and four to the right.
   d. With hands behind your back drop your head and lean down as far as you can. Keep your knees as straight as possible and raise your hands behind you.
   e. Hold for eight to ten seconds.
   f. Release your hands, reach down as low on your legs as you can, grasp your legs and pull gently.
   g. Hold for eight to ten seconds, bend your knees and stand up.
   h. Shake your arms and legs out.

Kneel on mat and place hands on mat as well (all fours).

8. Pectoral stretch.

   a. Move your hands forward (1 foot) on the mats.

   b. Slowly move your hips back and lower your chest and shoulders toward the mat while keeping your arms straight.

   c. Hold for eight to ten seconds and release.

   d. Slowly move your hips forward and down toward the mat.

   e. While keeping your arms straight look up toward the ceiling.

   f. Hold for eight to ten seconds and release.

9. Cat back.

   a. Round your back like a cat, drop your head at the same time.

   b. Hold for eight to ten seconds and slowly release.

   c. Then arch your back by bringing your head up and forming a U with your spine.

   d. Hold for eight to ten seconds and slowly release.

Kneel and keep waist and back straight.

10. Windmills.

    a. With your arms reaching out to the sides lean to left. Put left hand as close to the floor as possible and right hand up. Then return and lean to the right.

    b. Repeat eight to ten times.

11. Trunk twists.

    a. With your arms reaching out to the sides turn to the left as far as possible and look behind, return and turn to the right.

    b. Repeat eight to ten times.

Sitting with legs out in front.

12. Torso twist.

   a. Take your right foot and place it on the floor just outside your bent left knee.

   b. Place your left elbow on the outside of your right thigh while placing your hand on the mat.

   c. Turn your head and shoulders to the right and look behind.

Be sure to keep your hips on the mat and your right knee upright.

   d. Hold for eight to ten seconds.

   e. Repeat to the opposite side.

Extend both legs forward.

13. Sit and reach.

   a. Move your chest toward your ankles while reaching as far down your legs as you can.

   b. Grasp your lower legs and pull gently.

   c. Hold for eight to ten seconds and slowly release.

Lie on back in bent knee position.

14. Hamstring stretch.

   a. Slide left leg down to straight leg position.

   b. Bring your right knee to your chest.

   c. Reach up, grasp your right leg and pull toward chest.

   d. Hold for eight to ten seconds and release.

   e. Extend your right leg upward until your knee is straight.

   f. Reach up, grasp your leg and pull gently toward your shoulders.

g. Hold for eight to ten seconds and release.

h. Slowly lower your right leg to the floor.

i. Repeat with left leg.

15. Slowly roll head to the left and hold for two to three seconds then roll to the right and hold for two to three seconds. Repeat two more times.

16. Slowly inhale and clench your hands (make a fist) as tight as possible, hold two to three seconds and exhale while releasing the hands.

17. Repeat step 15.

18. Slowly inhale and raise your shoulders toward your ears, hold for two to three seconds and exhale while releasing the shoulders.

19. Repeat step 15.

20. Slowly inhale, hold for two to three seconds and then exhale.

This program implies access to a gym or a health club with Universal or Nautilus equipment. It also implies some kind of assistance or supervision. You can use free weights with which you'll definitely require the help of a "spotter."

A CWT program requires that you perform some kind of aerobic activity between stations. This could be rope jumping, running in place, riding an exercise bike or anything that will increase the heart rate. As noted, CWT activity, done properly, can contribute to aerobic fitness. You can, of course, use a progressive resistance machine or free weights without the intervening exercise and without the aerobic benefit.

There are many types of lifts and weight exercises you can engage in. For century riders and long-distance tourists, the emphasis should be on high repetitions (13 to 15) and not maximum weight, particularly if you are interested in building endurance.

Norman Sheil, past coach of the Canadian and British cycling teams, outlines a beginner or basic weight training program to help you build your strength and endurance for the coming season. Of course, you can build on it throughout the year and probably should if you want the full benefits, but that is beyond the province of this book.

Consider the following program designed by Sheil to complement or supplement the previous CWT program. While you can certainly perform these routines without assistance, I recommend that you do not do so. Weight training offers real benefits, but it should not be undertaken lightly. If at all possible do your weight training in a supervised setting.

BEGINNER'S TRAINING PROGRAM

	Repetitions		
	Set 1	Set 2	Set 3
Squat	15	12	10
Pullover	15	15	15
Dips	12	10	8
Upright Rowing	12	10	8
Bench Press	12	10	8
Bent-over Rowing	12	10	8
Press Behind Neck	12	10	8
Curl	12	10	8
Hyperextensions	15	15	15
Sit-ups	15	15	15

You should perform each exercise in turn until one set is completed, then the second set and, if possible, a third set. Try to move quickly from one exercise or set.

Concentrate on technique and complete the program briskly as you would in CWT, so you improve your cardiorespiratory fitness.

The amount of weight used will vary with each individual and will involve some trial and error. As a rule of thumb, begin by using one-eighth to one-fourth of body weight for all upper body exercises with the exception of straight arm pullovers which will require only an empty bar. For trunk exercises use about one-half of body weight and for squats begin with about three-quarters of body weight. To begin, remember that it is better to use lighter weights. You should increase weights by five-pound increments for arms and by ten-pound for trunk and legs. The correct weight will allow you to complete each exercise for the stated number of repetitions with maximum effort on the last two or three reps.

The objective of weight training is to maintain an overload situation. When it becomes possible to perform at least two more repetitions than recommended, increase the load for the next workout.

Example: Curl   Set 1 x 12 reps completed
                          Set 2 x 10 reps completed
                          Set 3 x 12 reps completed

The target for the third set was eight reps and 12 were performed, therefore increase the load by five pounds for the next workout. If fewer than ten repetitions had been performed the weight would remain unchanged.

Squat. Upright standing position with bar resting on shoulders at the back of the neck. Keeping the back straight and chest high, bend at knees and hips until thighs are parallel to the floor. Push up to starting position, using the large muscle groups in the hips. Avoid excessive forward movement of the knees by distributing weight on the heels as well as the balls of the feet.

Practice the full squat position with no bar, using a wall for assistance to learn balance.

Development: hips, thigh, lower back, chest.

Note: Squats must be performed with at least one spotter.

Straight Arm Pullover.

Lying on your back, hands shoulder-width apart, arms stretched fully over head. After inhaling fully, pull bar to the position directly over the chest, exhaling as the weight rises in an arc. Keep arms straight throughout.

Development: chest expansion, shoulder flexibility.

Dips.

Hands on chairs approximately shoulder width, arms straight. Legs extended to the front, chest high throughout the movement. Lower your body by bending at the elbows until upper arms are parallel to the floor. Press straight up to starting position.

Development: arms, shoulders, chest.

Upright Rowing.

Start in an erect standing position, with weight across the thighs. Feet are approximately hip-width apart, with hands close together.

Pull up along the abdomen and chest until bar reaches chin level. Keep elbows higher than the bar throughout the movement. The legs and body remain straight throughout the exercise.

Development: shoulders, upper back, arms.

Bench Press.

Lie on your back, hands gripping the bar slightly wider than shoulders with feet flat on the floor.

Starting at arm's length, bar about eye level, arch your

back so chest is high (hips still in contact with the bench). Lower bar to the center of the chest (under control) and press up and slightly back to starting position.

Development: chest, shoulders, arms.

Note: This exercise must be performed with a spotter.

Bent-over Rowing.   Feet are shoulder-width apart, hands slightly wider. With back straight and flat, bend forward at the waist until upper body is nearly parallel to the floor. Allow the legs to bend slightly.

Without any motion of the legs or torso, pull the bar up to touch at the bottom of the chest. Lower the bar under control to maintain body position.

Development: chest, shoulders, upper back.

Press Behind the Neck.   Stand upright with bar resting on shoulders at the back of the neck. Hand grip is slightly wider than shoulders.

Push bar to fully extend arms overhead. Lower weight to starting position avoiding movement of the legs and torso.

Development: shoulders and arms.

Curl.   Stand erect, hands gripping the bar at shoulder width, palms away from the body. Start in hand position, arms fully extended, bar resting on the thighs. Raise the bar to the chest, bending the arms at the elbow. Bar moves in an arc as the elbows remain at the sides.

Stand as straight as possible to limit the action to the arms.

Development: arms.

Back Hyperextension.   Lie facedown with hips elevated four to six inches above the floor (use padded boards or pillows). Hands placed behind the head with an assistant holding down the ankles and hips.

From starting position, arch back as far as possible, hold for one count, then lower head and torso to original position. The emphasis in this exercise is on complete contraction of the lower back muscles.

Sit-ups.   Lie on your back with knees bent, feet flat and close to the hips. Place hands on hips.

Tuck chin to chest and curl upper body up until chest touches the knees.

Development: abdominals.

Note: If you have any history of back problems, consult your physician first.

As I noted earlier, weight training should be undertaken in a controlled environment, particularly if you are working with free weights. Properly practiced, weight training can add much to your cycling and total fitness.

John N. Fetick, age 55, of Baltimore, Maryland, informs me that his

> weight training has shifted in partial interest from mere muscle toning to preparation for cycling. For instance, leg exercises done in the gym have proved invaluable when boarding the bike. Squatting with weights has provided a strong butt, knees and legs to perform on the bike. Endurance gained in weight training has helped to develop capacity in riding the bicycle. Even the principle of gradual weight increase to prevent soreness of the muscles has carried over to gradual lengthening of time spent on the bike: short, half-hour trips around the neighborhood back streets to break in the bicycle have now increased to longer trips. Severity of climbs has increased.

More and more recreational cyclists are engaging in some kind of weight training because the strength gained can make your cycling easier and more enjoyable.

I have found that weight training, with or without an aerobic emphasis, has helped me in the early season. I have particularly noted that when I engage in CWT in the late winter or early spring, I have fewer back, shoulder, and arm aches when I get back out on the road in March. I do a lot of hill climbing and have found even moderate, high-repetition weight training has made me stronger on the hills. Furthermore, I've found that the quadriceps exercises help me get up to steam quicker in the season. However, weight work does not mean you can skip any of the high-rpm, low-gear riding that will give you your base mileage.

American cycling coaches have come late to the belief that cyclists need more than cycling to improve their performance. We are slowly learning what the Eastern Bloc nations have known for years. Similarly, recreational cyclists are discovering that weight training can make them more powerful. Beyond that, there's a movement afoot in this country which I called the "total fitness movement," which is the inclination of athletes to cross-over and participate in other activities to help them achieve a full body fitness.

CROSS-TRAINING

America seems to be entering a new phase of participant sports. I think special interest activities will always remain and people will still have a favorite sport. On the other hand, with greater emphasis being placed on full body fitness, more attention is being given to cross-training—participating or competing in a number of compatible cardiovascular activities.

For the average, recreational athlete, cross-training has a number of distinct benefits. Assuming your primary activity is cycling, you might like to take some time off in the winter, simply as a change of pace, much like many amateur and professional racers. No matter how much we love a sport, most of us can benefit from time away from it.

Cross-training is a fine way to anticipate or prevent overuse injuries, which are not usually associated with cycling. However, I do know many runners who have switched to cycling while recuperating and now make it a regular part of their exercise routine, particularly in the summer when some people consider it too hot to run.

From a strictly physiological point of view it makes some sense to consider some kind of cross-training. You know that when you ride, you invoke a great deal of muscle activity, though the quadriceps show the most involvement and development. When you run, you involve different muscles, primarily the hamstrings and the shins. It stands to reason that when you are exercising both the front and back of the legs, you will be less likely to experience tendonitis and ligament damage.

Many cyclists engage in cross-training in the winter because they cannot ride or simply want some time off the bike. But this is true in many sports. Beth and Eric Heiden, who won so many medals in speed skating during the 1980 Olympics, cycled in the off-season to stay in shape. For them, this kind of training worked out very well. Beth went on to win the World Championship road race in 1980; Eric has become a professional bike racer.

Physiologists and coaches generally recommend that elite athletes should not engage in cross-training. For example, Stan Lindstedt, Ph.D., a muscle physiologist at the University of Wyoming, has performed muscle biopsies on cyclists who specialize in riding time trials. He compared these results with biopsies of marathon runners and concluded that, "It's hard to see what an athlete like a time-trialist would gain in terms of physical improvement by taking up running, even at a marathon level."

But for the recreational cyclist it's entirely another

matter. More important than optimum muscle activity—on the chemical level—is our ability to stay fit, stay healthy and stay interested. And cross-training can help in that regard.

For your cross-training you might add a weight program, as outlined earlier. Cross-country skiing and speed skating are very compatible with cycling, though facilities are not always available. A swimming program, three to four times a week for 30 to 40 minutes would provide a comparable workout, though it doesn't do much for the legs. Keep in mind that the best "test" of the cardiovascular benefit of an exercise is whether it will raise your pulse rate and keep it up for the prescribed period.

Jumping rope three or four times a week is a good exercise though I suspect you will find it more of a cold or rainy weather diversion than a complementary activity. I find it especially useful when I travel. There's only so much you can do in a motel room.

For compatibility and convenience, a maintenance running program is probably your best way to stay in shape in the off-season, unless for musculoskeletal reasons, running just isn't for you. If you want to run, ease into a program as outlined earlier in this chapter. Remember you are working different muscles in your legs, and though your heart is ready, they are not.

I'm assuming your primary objective is fitness—not to be an Olympic-caliber racer. Therefore, you want to control your weight, pulse, and blood pressure. To do that you would have to run at least four times a week for a minimum of thirty minutes each time.

I recall asking the great Belgian racer Eddy Merckx whether he did any weight work. He seemed amused by the question and answered through a translator that he didn't need big arms to pull him up the hills. No, the lack of weight training did not prevent Merckx from becoming the greatest professional cyclist of the century.

But for mere mortals, complementary exercises and training provide a balance, both physically and psychologically. Because of this interest in multiple sports participation, an entirely new sports category has arisen involving cycling, running, and swimming. The Triathlon, which originated in Hawaii, has filtered down to the other forty-nine states in a more modest form. In fact, mini-triathlon and biathlons are within the province of most well-conditioned cyclists.

Biathlons, sometimes called "half and wholes," calling for a 13-mile run and a 26-mile cycling leg, are quite common in many communities across the country and seem to draw an equal number of runners and cyclists. At these relatively short distances you would not need much specialized training in order to participate, especially if the event occurs in the fall as many do. I have participated in biathlons of this kind and find that a season of training as outlined in this book, plus a maintenance running program, makes me reasonably competitive. That means in addition to my cycling mileage I would run at least three times a week, two months before I am to compete. More often than not, these events are staged as cooperative ventures by local cycling and running clubs and have a distinct social dimension.

To participate in a full-scale triathlon (2.4-mile swim 112-mile bike ride, 26-mile run) is another matter entirely and involves starting your program as much as a full year before the event, at which time you would already have a solid cycling schedule. Nine months before the triathlon you should be running at least three times a week up to five miles each session. You should also swim one-quarter to one-half mile once or twice a week. In addition to your regular short cycling trips you should get in at least one long weekend ride of 70 to 90 miles. With six months to go you should have mastered this schedule.

For the next three months increase your running to at

least four times a week and your distance to six to eight miles. Now you will be swimming three times a week, anywhere from one half to one mile, preferably in the ocean or rough waters. You should be cycling no less than four to five times a week with one long ride of over 100 miles.

During the last three months you should be increasing your distances and frequencies in all events. You should run at least four times a week with some long runs in the 10-to-15-mile range and a 20-mile run a couple of weeks before the triathlon. If you ride your long distances on the weekend, run long during the middle of the week so you can balance your hard training days. You should swim at least three times a week with one swim up to a mile and a half. Cycling mileage should be 200 to 250.

Try to compete in biathlons and mini-triathlons during the last months to get the feel of doing these events in tandem.

The above sketch is not meant as a training schedule— there are magazines and books devoted to that subject; I simply wanted to give you some idea of a minimum amount of training you'd have to undertake to participate in a full triathlon. If you have time and the inclination, a triathlon is the ultimate test of your total fitness. But if all you can manage is a shortened form of the real thing, that is equally good because it will still put you on an accelerated fitness program that will add another dimension to your cycling. Small-scale biathlons and triathlons are being held all over the country and involve training and distance well within the province of a fit cyclist. I encourage you to participate.

Staying Healthy

I would like to think this chapter is both redundant and necessary. Redundant if you do everything right, necessary if you don't. The fact of the matter is that cycling is a very safe activity that is particularly kind to weight-bearing joints. While I have no bone to pick with running, I don't see the layoffs due to injuries in cycling that I know occur in running. I haven't seen any formal study with comparable results but one would be very useful.

Let's consider the flip side of the coin for a minute. Not only does cycling *not* induce injuries, it helps those with injuries come back to health and sometimes full mobility. There cannot be a better testimonial to the efficacy of an activity.

One tenet of this book is that literally everyone, no matter his or her level of fitness or degree of infirmity, can benefit greatly from the use of the bike in a sensible, developmental fitness program. I have in front of me dozens of personal fitness stories from cyclists who have used biking as therapy, particularly for back injuries. While these examples do not constitute medical endorsements, they do dramatize the benefit of cycling as therapy.

Thomas C. Yantz, age 40, of Colonia, New Jersey, injured his back while helping to dock an oil tanker at a large refinery, an injury that was aggravated by his being about 40 pounds overweight. Aware that John Marino, ultramarathon cyclist and past holder of the cross-country record, had used cycling to help him overcome a back injury, Yantz tried the same thing. In three months of cycling he lost 32 pounds and noticed the pain in his back had "practically disappeared. As long as I ride at least 100 miles per week I have no trouble with my back. But if I stop riding for a week or more, the pain returns."

While stationed in Europe with the Army, Bill Greene of Killeen, Texas, enjoyed running and participated in 10ks. During a run he pulled his left hamstring and the leg did not respond until he had a disc surgically removed. The nerve damage affected his gait and he could no longer run efficiently. In a year he put on an extra 35 pounds. So as an experiment Greene "cleaned up an old 3-speed and pedaled around the neighborhood for about 20 minutes two or three times a week." He is now riding centuries and has never felt better.

Cycling can also help bring individuals back to health from debilitating injuries. William Caldwell of Madison, Wisconsin, was injured in a motorcycle accident that broke both femurs, crushed his right patella, separated the left knee, and fractured the left tibia. The paroneal nerves in both legs were damaged resulting in "foot drop." Prognosis: He might not walk again.

After five operations he could walk with pain. Following more surgery his doctor recommended swimming, weight training and cycling, and he particularly embraced the latter, participating in one 40-mile ride in a leg cast. He has now developed a training schedule which includes interval training, long rides (75 miles), short time trials (25 miles) and easy recovery days. He notes that a remarkable thing happened. "As my legs became stronger the pain I had experienced in varying degrees for nine years disappeared. I was pain free and for the first time since the wreck I was proud of my legs. My bicycling has given me back my life or at least has enabled me to truly enjoy it."

Certain thematic threads run through all these stories. Many people recovering from all types of injuries embrace cycling because it is easy. Furthermore, it is gentle and rhythmic with no jarring of the weight-bearing joints. Cycling is especially kind to the back and the knees, two injury-prone areas for countless Americans. Although the stories I'm offering are demonstrably anecdotal, I hope they both encourage you the reader and persuade the medical community to take a long, hard look at the efficacy of cycling as therapy. With guidance and restraint, hundreds of thousands of Americans suffering from back, knee and other problems might be able to participate in aerobic exercise which can help heal the body and the spirit.

If cycling heals, it can also hurt. And it usually hurts if your bike isn't set up right, you're lugging too big a gear, or you're overzealous in your training. Personally, my only injury from cycling is when I took a spill. Bad as it was I was back to cycling in three days, before I could walk properly.

The advice in this chapter is my own and in my own words, though I can't help but be influenced by Drs. Eugene Gaston and David Smith, cyclists and medical correspondents who have been providing state-of-the-art medical advice to readers of *Bicycling* magazine and others for the last decade. In their own right they have saved a lot of heads and necks. My advice here is meant to be anecdotal as I address problems associated with incorrect bike setup or poor usage. If you have structural problems, see your doctor.

Earlier in this book I spent a great deal of time on bicycle setup, demonstrating that an improperly set-up bike could lead to all sorts of problems. If your saddle is too high or low, you could develop pain in the knees. If too high, you will be reaching for the pedals at the bottom of the downstroke, stretching your leg and awkwardly engaging your hip. Riding with a low saddle will not permit you to extend and fully engage your powerful thigh muscles. Reaching out for a too-long stem could have a deleterious effect on your back and shoulder muscles.

So a lot of problems can be caught early if your bike is set up properly and if you're using the right equipment.

Most beginner cyclists experience some discomfort in the neck, back, shoulders, buttocks, wrists and hands. Usually, time in the saddle will take care of most of these problems. As suggested, you probably should put some kind of foam padding on your handlebars to help cushion the road shock. I've found that makes an awful lot of difference, particularly when cycling moderate to long distances. Your bike shops offer a number of brands and will put it on for a small fee.

Saddle Problems.   I have seen people put foam padding on their saddles midway into a ride to make the journey home a little easier. That is not a very good idea as the practice just robs you of energy. For most people, spending time in the saddle will help condition the rear end. Unfortunately, you don't know whether you will like a saddle until it's been on your bike for some time. Saddles come in leather and vinyl. Conventional logic says that over time—much time—a leather saddle will shape to you. That will not happen with a vinyl saddle whose advantage is that it's a little more comfortable to begin with.

For women there are special anatomical considerations. The bicycle industry has been shamefully slow in responding to the legitimate needs of women and still designs bikes for the standard American male. There are saddles, such as Avocet and the Brooks B-72 that have been designed for a woman's larger pelvic structure and more options are becoming available. You should carefully check the fit of the saddle at purchase. Or you might consider upgrading your saddle to one especially designed for women.

I have already noted that many off-the-rack bikes don't fit prospective female cyclists and frequently the gearing is high. These same bikes often come with stems that are too long and handlebars that are too wide. Since you won't grow into a bike, it is essential that women and all cyclists start with a bike that fits. That is the best defense against pain and suffering.

Ultimately, saddles are a very personal choice and cause some very personal problems, such as saddle soreness and numb crotch. Even after the breaking-in period, some riders still experience some of these maladies. If you are in this category you might have to experiment with saddles, trying one of the "grooved" varieties such as the Avocet Touring or Selle Royal.

Also check the tilt of the saddle. You will experience excess pressure on the perineum if your saddle is tilted too far backward or forward. In such circumstances a micro-adjusting seatpost is very handy as a fraction of an inch in tilt or fore-and-aft adjustment can make a lot of difference.

New riders sometimes experience saddle soreness and irritation because of the shorts or underpants (or both) they wear. Some seams and your movement in the saddle will eventually cause irritation, perhaps saddle sores and blisters. You can probably prevent this problem by riding in seam-less cycling shorts. Men usually don't wear undershorts; for hygienic reasons, women usually do. Either way it is important to keep your cycling shorts free of bacteria. That means washing them frequently—and having a spare set.

To cut down on friction and possible irritation many

cyclists put Vaseline or cornstarch on their buttocks and genital area before long rides. This seems to help. But again, proper hygiene is essential.

Over the years men have complained about cycling irritating (or causing) prostate problems. There is no strong medical evidence that cycling hurts or helps the prostate, though if you are having trouble experiment with a grooved saddle and with the tilt.

A few male cyclists have reported that following long rides, they are unable to have an erection. No one knows the reasons for this and whether the malady is widespread, which I doubt. If you are having this problem and think it's associated with cycling, you might try some of the recommendations outlined in the saddle section. See a urologist to determine whether the bladder or prostate is involved. A final solution is to lay off cycling.

For those who continue to experience saddle soreness or discomfort after trying all the preceding strategies, you might try other options such as the Bummer or the Dan Henry sling. The former is commercially available; the latter you can make based on plans published by Dan Henry and available through *Bicycling* magazine.

With the interest in cycling much research and development is being devoted to the question of saddle comfort. This includes more choices in anatomical saddles as well as in various saddle coverings. I'm presently testing a saddle covering made of synthetic fat, material used in the bedding of burn patients. Unnamed as of now, it seems quite comfortable and will be on the market by the time this book is published and available through retail bike shops.

Other commercial options are available, such as the Coveralls® brands manufactured by Grab On and available at retail. Easy Seat® offers a kind of dual seat that is designed to support both sides of your pelvic bone. A look at a recent issue of *Bicycling* magazine will provide numerous alternatives for individuals not well served by traditional bicycle saddles.

Numbness in the Foot. I have written about the biomechanics of cycling, the relationship between the body and the bike. Needless to say, if the bicycle doesn't fit the body or the two are joined improperly at the key locations, irritation or injury will occur.

Where your foot is attached to the pedals is an important biomechanical pressure point. You can avoid foot problems if you take a few precautions. Fortunately, foot problems don't seem to be a major problem for cyclists, though numb feet seem to plague many beginners.

You cannot do the kind of cycling I'm advising in tennis and jogging shoes. The shank is not stiff enough and sooner or later you will feel the pressure of the pedal on the sole of your foot, particularly as you increase your mileage. Cycling shoes will not only position you properly over the pedals, they will absorb some of the stresses associated with pedaling. You will recall that there is no *best* cycling shoe, though some of the touring shoes are very flexible and have shanks that really do not soak up much stress.

I sometimes experience numbness in my strong foot (leg) after some hard cycling. My remedy is to loosen the toe straps. I'm told by racers that they don't usually experience this problem because they consciously pull up on the pedals, relieving some of the pressure. Foot numbness is also associated with pushing too hard on the pedals in too high a gear. A brisk cadence should help.

You might experience some irritation of the toes. This could be due to your toes (and the front of the shoe) rubbing against the toe clips. Check and see whether there's enough clearance between shoe and toe clip.

Some cyclists wear socks, some don't; it's a personal preference. Whatever your choice, good hygiene should prevail. I usually don't wear socks and before I ride I spread cornstarch or Vaseline on my feet. Messy, but seems to prevent blisters. (Yes, I wash well after a ride.)

While there are changes in the marketplace, cycling shoes have traditionally been narrow, which has been a problem for cyclists, especially those with wide feet. Make sure you are not stuffing your foot into a little Italian shoe.

Sometimes numbness of the foot can be remedied by switching to a narrow platform pedal, such as the Lyotard or Barelli, which leaves the outside of your foot free of pedal pressure.

Usually, numb feet in cycling are associated with usage. If you improve your technique and modify your equipment, the problem should be resolved. Please keep in mind that all numb feet or poor circulation is not necessarily caused by cycling. If the problem persists, you should see your doctor.

More prevalent than the numb foot syndrome are problems associated with the knee. However, with proper bike setup, wide-range gearing and sensible cycling, you will probably not experience any discomfort in the knee. After all, one of the great attractions of cycling is that it puts no pressure on the weight-bearing joints.

Knee Problems.   Most sports medicine doctors, trainers and experienced riders agree that knee injuries are usually associated with technique. Inexperienced cyclists, often feeling good, push high gears before their muscles, ligaments, and tendons are strong enough, especially early in the season. As I've said before, a brisk pedal cadence is the best technique all through the seasons. Big gears are a trap and a danger.

During the writing of this book I gave up my bike for a few days to have the components replaced and used a racing bike for a week. After a few days I noticed my knees were getting sore. Though it was mid-season and I had in a lot of base miles, I wasn't used to climbing hills in a 52-inch gear, which was the lowest selection on this racing bike. I wasn't prepared for that. When I stopped using the bike, the pain in my knees went away.

William Farrell, Director of the New England Cycling Academy, has found that some knee pain is associated with cleat placement. He suggested that the following conditions must be met: "the ball of the foot should be positioned over the pedal spindle; the shoe must also be mounted with careful consideraton of the natural inward or outward rotation of the cyclist's hop and knee." If you have eliminated the more obvious reasons for knee pain, check the fore-aft and rotational adjustment of your toe clip, keeping in mind Farrell's rule of thumb.

By some estimates 80 to 90 percent of new riders probably put their seats up too high, which stretches the knees unnaturally. Often these riders will move the seat forward so they are closer to the handlebars, but that does very little for the knees.

Again, proper setup and technique will likely keep you immune from most knee problems. However, if you still experience pain, stop cycling and see a podiatrist or a sports medicine doctor. In his examination of 23 elite National cyclists podiatrist Mitchell Feingold discovered a large percentage of them had abnormal foot functions and recommended that nine of the group be fitted with rigid orthotics, a casted piece of plastic that helps stabilize the foot and reduce stress. An orthotic helps stabilize the foot and puts it in a better relationship to the pedal. This might be a consideration for you.

Feingold also found that most of the riders he tested were not very flexible and put them on stretching programs to increase flexibility of the lower extremities. To reduce your chance of injury and pulled muscles, you should do regular stretching exercises, such as outlined in the previous chapter. You should also take time to warm up and cool down sufficiently.

Jeff Paulsen, medical director of the Coors Classic stage race, has found that among competitive cyclists the most frequent cause of joint, soft-tissue, and ligament pain is significant increases in training distance and speed. Since distance and speed are relative, Paulsen's advice also applies to recreational cyclists.

He suggests that low-gear training (below 70 inches), stretching and weight work will help you get started with little discomfort. All the more reason to include these procedures in your off-season total fitness program.

Back Pain.   I noted earlier that a number of people with back complaints have successfully taken up cycling. On the other hand, people who cycle sometimes experience backaches, which usually disappear with time in the saddle and a regimen of stretching exercises. If the ache persists, you should move the saddle forward slightly as it should help unkink the lower back. At the same time you will probably have to raise the saddle a little and tilt it backward slightly. If your stem is too long that could be the reason for your discomfort.

You might experience some pain in the shoulder blades and neck area. If these don't go away with time in the saddle, check the distance between your set of the handlebars; you could be reaching too far. For the neck pain you might try keeping your neck down but eyes up, raising the handlebars slightly or switching to another kind called randoneur bars which don't have as much drop. Or you might want to switch to regular upright bars. Use what gives you the most comfort. Speed is less important if you are in pain.

One way to alleviate lower back pain is to do some gentle stretches before and after cycling. Here's an easy one: Lie facing the floor and raise yourself with your forearms, while gently arching your back. This relieves fatigue.

I've already touched on remedies for sore wrists and hands: Handlebar padding and cycling gloves often provide relief. As recommended earlier, you should try to periodically change the position of your hands on the bars. Check the distance from the seat to the handlebars. For the average person the distance should be equal to the length of the rider's forearm from elbow to fingertips. Be careful with that rule of thumb as it will not apply to a lot of riders.

Numb hands and fingers have been associated with cycling in cold weather. The best remedy is to wear padded gloves when the temperature gets 50°F. or lower if you're particularly susceptible. I use ski gloves during the cool months and find they work very well.

Almost all "user-related" problems can be prevented through proper bike fit, setup and use. If the bike fits, you should experience very little discomfort after the initial breaking-in period. If you put in your base miles with prudence and restraint, staying out of the big gears until your muscles, tendons, and ligaments can handle them, knee problems, the bane of so many other sports, should not trouble you.

But staying healthy assumes much more. Most of the time you will be cycling in an environment populated by cars. To remain healthy you have to obey all the rules of the road and common driver courtesy. Remember, you are a driver of a vehicle with all attendant rights and responsibilities. You have to read the road and be able to anticipate trouble spots. You must develop a kind of sixth sense in traffic that tells you when a car door is going to open. When riding with other cyclists, particularly ones you don't know, get a handle on their habits right away and stay far in front of nervous riders and those that brake at every opportunity. Don't follow or overlap another rider's wheel unless you know his or her habits very well. Always wear a hard-shell helmet. If you find yourself going down, tuck your head in and try to roll through on the back of your shoulder. Don't try to stiff arm the road; you'll likely break your wrist.

Most falls are not serious. While writing this book I took a spill as I rode at a good clip, falling on my thigh and shoulder. I stopped for ice and peroxide for the road rash and cycled twenty miles home. But I was sore the next couple of days. Interestingly, I was back cycling before I could walk briskly and run, which demonstrates the therapeutic effect of cycling on a badly bruised hip.

If sometimes we are not gentle on the bike, the bike is almost always gentle on our bodies. Numerous women report cycling well into pregnancies. I know cyclists who have ridden up to the ninth month of pregnancy with their doctors' approval. They report relatively easy deliveries because of the exercise and most were back on the bike within three weeks. From watching my wife exercise through two pregnancies, I believe cycling, indoors or outside, is a good idea and urge physiologists to conduct controlled tests on cycling during pregnancy.

The Added Dimension

While conducting research for this book, I talked to and corresponded with hundreds of people across the country. Some are Olympic-caliber racers; most are men and women who have successfully used the bicycle as a fitness tool.

That term, that claim, can be very misleading. In the preceding chapter I've referred to racers going up to 40 mph and individuals who can barely straddle the frame and mount the bike, yet all are getting fitter through cycling.

I've followed the racing circuit for about seven years and have been familiar with the brilliance of our amateur cyclists, who are just beginning to get the recognition they deserve.

What surprised me in my research is how many *average* people have turned to cycling as a kind of therapy. I have recounted some stories; there are many others, equally interesting. I've interviewed individuals who have used the bike to help them overcome addiction to dope and alcohol. Others, so deeply controlled by depression, found genuine salvation in the bike. A woman who had been fighting a nine-year battle with anorexia needed "something that would provide exercise to burn some of the extra calories that I hoped to allow myself to ingest. I also needed something that would provide a bit of self-confidence." She added that "on the first day that I biked an extra hour in the early morning before work I actually felt hungry during the day. This was a major accomplishment for someone who had lost, denied, and disregarded such cues for so long."

A 29-year-old man from Brookfield, Massachusetts, had a marijuana habit for twelve years. His raging appetite brought his weight up to 230 pounds. After hearing all the cures from numerous doctors, he started cycling and remarks that

> this may sound like an exaggerated overstatement, but the bicycle was my salvation. Cycling has turned my life around. It has changed my life-style, cured my physical ills, and most important has given me an aid for my mind.
>
> When I first started riding, I would go five or six miles and I thought I was doing great. Being obese all my life, this liberty of self-locomotion was a great feeling and boy could I fly down those hills. As anyone who gets into cycling soon discovers, the more you ride the more you want to ride. If you can ride five miles, can you ride ten? When you ride ten, can you ride twenty? When you ride twenty miles for the first time you feel proud of your seemingly superhuman feat and then wonder just what your limits are.

This reborn cyclist has already lost 40 pounds and is closing in on 175. His resting pulse is 60, down from 78. His immune system has improved considerably. He is, in his own words, a "new man."

There must be millions of Americans on regular medication. Certainly many take medication for various forms of arthritis. Not Mrs. Carroll Arnold, age 60, of Sumner, Washington, who was fortunate to find a doctor who recommended cycling for her arthritis of the knee, which made even walking very painful. One year later she reports that through regular cycling, "Not only did I get a lot of enjoyment, the knee got better, pain went away and I could walk in comfort. I also lost weight. I have more energy and am more fit than I've been in years." (Her husband, who had been taking medication to regulate his heart, improved his condition so much through cycling that his doctor took him off medication.)

If cycling reaches back and, therapeutically, brings people to health, it also anticipates the fitness needs of a growing body of citizens, particularly women. American female cyclists are the very best amateurs in the world and the likes of Sue Novara-Reber, Sheila Young, Beth Heiden and Rebecca Twigg have dominated the international competitive scene for the last decade. These champions are just beginning to bring their sisters to the sport.

Lorraine Williams of Lawrenceburg, Indiana, used to be an enthusiastic bystander, cheering on the men in her life, until she found the bicycle, until she found herself. This is her story:

Now, you wouldn't exactly group me with the likes of Len Halderman or Rebecca Twigg or even your neighborhood Senior IV racer. You might even pass me quite easily on the next steep hill. But it doesn't matter. You see, cycling has made me realize that I am an athlete anyway. No matter how fast or how far I can ride, I'm out there doing it. *My* legs are pushing and pulling those pedals. *My* lungs are huffing up the hills. *My* ego makes me tough out a 210 mile tour in weather in which only two years ago I wouldn't have walked to the grocery store.

But it's been a long haul in a short time. Previous to this new sense of myself as physically acceptable, I was solely an enthusiastic bystander. In grade school

I cheered for my brothers playing Little League baseball. In junior high and high school the brothers changed to boyfriends, but I still cheered from the sidelines.

There wasn't really a whole lot of choice in my small school, even as recently as the mid-seventies. Besides cheerleading, the only sports for girls were struggling basketball and track teams. Since cheerleaders were generally assured of more dates than basketball players, I went the cheerleader route.

I do, however, distinctly remember trying track one year. Shin splints and occasional third place finishes were not enough encouragement for me to continue my athletic career. The coach agreed.

The college scene wasn't much better. Having an already firmly established image of the nonathletic me, I didn't push for embarrassment. Instead, I pushed myself in academics and gazed wistfully at the red and white plaid skirts of the field hockey team or my roommate bouncing off to sorority volleyball. Then I reminded myself that I "wasn't good in sports" and went to the library.

Meanwhile, I furtively satisfied my ego with running a few miles (early in the morning so no *real* runner would see me), swimming a couple of laps, or riding my bike around campus. I was your basic clandestine athlete, longing for an Athletic Accomplishment to make me legitimate. After all, athletics means *competitive* sports, doesn't it? And I was afraid to compete.

Perhaps this fear of losing began sometime during my long association with athletic achievers. My vicarious participation in the sporting world, begun with my brothers, progressed to the school jock—standout in football, basketball, and of course, track. Number two serious relationship reinforced my inferiority in running, waterskiing, and even bowling. Then a couple of college football players came along. More enthusiastic bystanding. So, of course I couldn't settle for Joe Walk-Around-The-Block-After-Dinner to marry. No sir, it was a marathoner, lifeguard, cross-country skier and bike racer that I chose for marital bliss.

He brought with him a whole shelf full of trophies and ribbons and medals to sustain my self-doubt. Then he promptly bought me a bike and, for the love of the sport, dragged me out on the roads day after day. And I, for the sake of love, went.

One year later, down some melting road in Findlay, Ohio, during the Hancock Horizontal Hundred, it dawned on me: I am in the middle of an Athletic Accomplishment. There amidst the dogs and the dust and the bugs, the heat and the wind and the saddle sores, I discovered that I was athletic after all. Riding 100 miles under seven and a half hours is a genuine, certifiable, athletic performance.

But, after 23 years, one wants to be absolutely sure about these things, so I put my shaky new self-image on the line. After a winter of sporadic training I found myself braving the elements of the Tour of the Scioto River Valley in Columbus, Ohio. All 210 miles of it. I considered the thought that it might be cheating to acquire an Athletic Accomplishment via tandem, but after ten miles or so of headwind battle, decided that it was probably acceptably difficult to merit the AA seal. When the cable broke, I was reasonably sure. By the end of the ride, I knew.

I also knew that I didn't have to bring home trophies and ribbons. I didn't need public acclaim or newspaper coverage. I didn't even need an Athletic Accomplishment. The status of athlete, I learned, is achieved by competing against myself. Every day that I am on the road or the rollers, enjoying it or not, I am becoming more athletic. Bicycling has given me a new, exciting perspective on my physical potential.

The sport is in the participation. The competition is in overcoming poor self-esteem.

And I'm winning.

Cycling is an equal opportunity fitness activity. Once conditioned, women perform remarkably well in the sport and are aided by having the greater part of their muscle mass concentrated in the legs.

The underlying premise of this book is that cycling is an ideal fitness activity, not only because it delivers all the vital cardiorespiratory benefits, but because it can be taken up by anyone, no matter his or her present level of fitness. Cycling will meet you in your present state.

Within cycling there is considerable variety. You can attain your prescribed level of fitness through touring, commuting, racing or fast recreational riding. You can join a club or go it alone. You can take long tours or short tours. You can cycle in this country or anywhere in the world.

You can become fit through some very utilitarian methods, such as cycling to work, school or on short trips around town. The key is frequency, not big mileage.

As you have seen, cycling can be an effective way to lose weight, control blood pressure and regulate heart rate. Certainly you should see your doctor before starting a vigorous program, but make sure he or she knows that other people have earned marvelous benefits from a regular cycling program. No doctor should argue with your desire to reduce medication through exercise.

Cycling can encourage a positive frame of mind, help overcome anxiety and depression. Seven years ago, Nancy A. Messinger of Seekonk, Massachusetts, fell off a horse and sustained a trimalleolar fracture of the right ankle and was informed that she would be in pain for the rest of her life. Her foot was held together with a plate, rod and screws. After a number of operations, including bone graft and electrical stimulation, she was in worse shape than before surgery and was on crutches.

Her migraines, which she had suffered from for twenty years, became worse, exacerbated by the pain in her leg. Depression set in. She gave up.

A year ago she went on a program of diet, exercise and meditation to relieve the migraines, lift the depression and heal the leg. With a great deal of guts and determination she recently rode her first century and literally burned her crutches. She writes that "as I pulled into the finish point nine hours and 42 minutes after the start I had tears in my eyes. I had done it. I was no longer a handicapped person, a cripple, but rather an accomplished cyclist. I am still so swell-headed that I can barely get my bike helmet on! I am learning how to live."

Nancy Messinger's triumph, echoed in the words "I am learning how to live," crystallizes the very essence of bicycling as a lifesport which delivers fitness, independence and peace of mind. That cycling makes you mobile in the largest sense implies you will cross landscapes under your own power and experience the exhilaration associated with genuine independence. There is a human dimension to cycling that will sustain you.

The anecdotal material in this book—the range of very moving success stories—to a certain extent runs ahead of conventional medical wisdom. And there's nothing wrong with the people showing the way. Perhaps there is a double benefit here: These stories will inspire you to excellence and also move the medical community to take a more sympathetic attitude toward bicycling.

I hope this book will inspire you to thoroughly embrace cycling as a fitness activity. Cycling can transform your life. And when it does, drop me a line. I'm anxious to hear about your successes.

Appendix

I Pulse Monitors

FINGER SENSOR UNITS

Pulse-Tach CPS4
The Sharper Image
300 Broadway
Suite 28
San Francisco, CA 94133

Genesis Exercise Computer
Biometric Systems, Inc.
4040 Del Ray Avenue
Marina Del Ray, CA 90291

Pulse Minder (no. 7719)
Computer Instruments Inc.
100 Madison Avenue
Hempstead, NY 11550

Novatec Pulse Rate Monitor
Nellie's Cardiac and Exercise Inc.
226 E. Las Tunas Drive
San Gabriel, CA 91775

EARLOBE SENSORS

Amerec PM-110
Amerec Corporation
P.O. Box 3825
Bellevue, WA 98009

Sears Digital Electronic Exercise/Pulse Monitor
Distributed by Sears

CHEST MONITORS

Exersentry Heart Rate Monitor
Respironics Inc.
650 Seco Road
Monroeville, PA 15146

Pacer 2000H
Veltec Inc.
P.O. Box 1156
Ft. Collins, CO 80522

II COMPUTERS

Cat Eye Cyclocomputer
Tsuyama Mfg. Co. Ltd.
2-8-25, Kuwazu
Higashi Sumiyoshi-ku
Osaka, Japan

Pacer 2000
Veltec, Inc.
P.O. Box 1156
Ft. Collins, CO 80522

Entex Bike Computer
National Sales Headquarters
15605 Carmenita Road
Santa Fe Springs, CA 90670

Push
Attivo Corporation
Box 852
Longmont, CA 80501

Velo Coach
Biotechnology Inc.
6924 NW 46 Street
Miami, FL 33166

Peugeot Sports Computer
Cycles Peugeot USA
Box 277
555 Gotham Parkway
Carlstadt, NJ 07072

Cyclotron
Calfax Inc.
15 E. 26 Street
New York, NY 10010

Cyclotronic
IKU
postbus 22
3417 zg Montfoort (u)
Holland
   (U.S. importer:
   Andrew Fisher Cycle Co.
   Inc.
   23 E. 26th Street
   New York, NY 10010)

Cyclometer 20
Avocet Inc.
Box 7615
Menlo Park, CA 94015

III Cycling Organizations

Bicycling Magazine
33 East Minor Street, Emmaus, PA 18049. (215) 967-5171.
The most widely circulated magazine of all aspects of
bicycling. Nine issues per year provide information on
touring, road tests and consumer guides, maintenance and
repair, cycling technique, commuting, racing, fitness and
more. Yearly subscription, $13.97. (U.S.)

American Youth Hostels (AYH)
National Administrative Office, 1332 I Street NW, Suite
800, Washington, DC 20005. (202) 783-6161.
AYH offers a network of hostels in the U.S. and 56 foreign
countries where bicycle tourists can stay for a few dollars.
Members receive the monthly newspaper *Hosteling*, which
prints a schedule of events and a handbook listing hostels
throughout the country. Cycling, hiking and skiing activities are offered, and AYH-led group bicycle tours can take
you all over the country and to almost anywhere in the
world.

Bicycle Federation
1055 Thomas Jefferson Street, NW, Suite 316, Washington,
DC 20007. (202) 337-3094.
Executive Director: Katie Moran. Established in 1977,
the Bicycle Federation is a nonprofit, national organization committed to increasing "the awareness, acceptance

and safe use of the bicycle as a mode of transportation."
An activist group.

Bicycle Forum
Box 8311, Missoula, MT 59807. (406) 728-4497.
Editor-in-Chief: John Williams. The Bicycle Forum is a
nonprofit organization devoted to advancing the state of
the art in bicycle program work. They put out a journal
and provide local bike program specialists and activists
with safety and encouragement materials.

Bicycle Manufacturers Association of America (BMA)
1101 Fifteenth Street, NW, Washington, DC 20005. (202)
452-1166.
James J. Hayes: contact. Leader in stimulating nationwide
interest in the development of bikeways and the promo-
tion of bike safety. Provides statistics on the bicycle
marketplace, industry trends, sales, etc.

Bikecentennial
P.O. Box 8308, Missoula, MT 59807. (406) 721-1776.
The national nonprofit service organization for touring
cyclists. Bikecentennial is the expert in giving cyclists all
the touring information they need. Provides resource guide,
bimonthly newsletter, etc.

League of American Wheelmen (LAW)
10 East Read Street, P.O. Box 988, Baltimore, MD 21203.
(301) 727-2022.
The League is the national nonprofit organization of bicyclists
that is dedicated to promoting the use of the bicycle and
protecting the rights of cyclists. Founded in 1880, the
LAW is not only the country's oldest bicycle federation,
but the leading advocacy group today for bicyclists who
are interested in touring, recreational riding and commuting.

Professional Racing Organization (PRO)
1524 Linden Street, Allentown, PA 18102. (215) 821-6862.

Jack Simes: President. Organization designed to represent and promote the professional category of athletes in competitive cycling.

United States Cycling Federation (USCF)
1750 East Boulder Street, Colorado Springs, CO 80909.
(303) 632-5551 ext. 281.
The governing body of competitive cycling in the U.S.

IV English Gear Chart for 27" Wheels

Rear Sprocket

Chainwheel	34	33	32	31	30	29	28	27	26	25	24	23	22	21	20	19	18	17	16	15	14	13	Chainwheel
34	27.0	27.8	28.6	29.6	30.6	31.6	32.7	34.0	35.3	36.7	38.2	39.9	41.7	43.7	45.9	48.3	51.0	54.0	57.3	61.2	65.5	70.6	34
35	27.8	28.6	29.5	30.5	31.5	32.5	33.7	35.0	36.3	37.8	39.3	41.0	42.9	45.0	47.2	49.7	52.5	55.5	59.0	63.0	67.5	71.9	35
36	28.6	29.45	30.4	31.4	32.4	33.5	34.7	36.0	37.3	38.8	40.5	42.2	44.1	46.2	48.6	51.1	54.0	57.1	60.7	64.8	69.4	74.7	36
37	29.4	30.3	31.2	32.2	33.3	34.4	35.6	37.0	38.4	40.0	41.6	43.4	45.4	47.5	50.0	52.5	55.5	58.7	62.4	66.6	71.3	76.8	37
38	30.2	31.1	32.1	33.1	34.2	35.3	36.6	38.0	39.4	41.0	42.7	44.6	46.6	48.8	51.3	54.0	57.0	60.3	64.1	68.4	73.2	78.9	38
39	31.0	31.9	32.9	34.0	35.1	36.3	37.6	39.0	40.5	42.1	43.9	45.8	47.9	50.1	52.6	55.4	58.5	61.9	65.8	70.2	75.2	81.0	39
40	31.8	32.7	33.8	34.8	36.0	37.2	38.5	40.0	41.5	43.2	45.0	47.0	49.1	51.4	54.0	56.8	60.0	63.5	67.5	72.0	77.1	83.0	40
41	32.6	33.5	34.6	35.7	36.9	38.1	39.5	41.0	42.4	44.2	46.1	48.1	50.3	52.7	55.3	58.2	61.5	65.1	69.1	73.8	79.0	85.1	41
42	33.4	34.4	35.4	36.6	37.8	39.1	40.5	42.0	43.6	45.3	47.2	49.3	51.5	54.0	56.7	59.6	63.0	66.7	70.8	75.6	81.0	87.2	42
43	34.1	35.2	36.3	37.5	38.7	40.0	41.4	43.0	44.6	46.4	48.3	50.4	52.8	55.2	58.0	61.1	64.5	68.2	72.5	77.4	82.9	89.3	43
44	34.9	36.0	37.1	38.3	39.6	40.9	42.4	44.0	45.7	47.5	49.5	51.6	54.0	56.6	59.4	62.5	66.0	69.9	74.3	79.2	84.9	91.3	44
45	35.7	36.8	38.0	39.2	40.5	41.8	43.4	45.0	46.7	48.6	50.7	52.9	55.2	57.9	60.8	63.9	67.5	71.5	76.0	81.0	86.7	93.4	45
46	36.5	37.6	38.8	40.1	41.4	42.8	44.4	46.0	47.8	49.7	51.8	54.0	56.5	59.1	62.1	65.3	69.0	73.1	77.6	82.7	88.7	95.5	46
47	37.3	38.5	39.7	40.9	42.3	43.7	45.3	47.0	48.8	50.8	52.9	55.3	57.5	60.4	63.4	66.8	70.5	74.6	79.3	84.6	90.6	97.6	47
48	38.1	39.3	40.5	41.8	43.2	44.6	46.2	48.0	49.9	51.8	54.0	56.3	58.7	61.7	64.8	68.2	72.0	76.2	81.0	86.4	92.6	99.6	48
49	38.9	40.1	41.3	42.7	44.1	45.6	47.2	49.0	50.9	52.9	55.1	57.5	60.1	63.0	66.2	69.6	73.5	77.8	82.7	88.2	94.5	101.7	49
50	39.7	40.9	42.2	43.5	45.0	46.5	48.2	50.0	51.9	54.0	56.2	58.7	61.3	64.3	67.5	71.0	75.0	79.4	84.4	90.0	96.4	103.8	50
51	40.5	41.7	43.0	44.4	45.9	47.4	49.1	51.0	53.0	55.1	57.3	59.8	62.6	65.5	68.8	72.5	76.5	81.0	86.1	91.8	98.4	108.0	51
52	41.3	42.5	43.9	45.3	46.8	48.4	50.1	52.0	54.0	56.2	58.5	61.0	63.8	66.9	70.2	73.9	78.0	82.6	87.8	93.6	100.3	108.0	52
53	42.1	43.4	44.7	46.2	47.7	49.3	51.1	53.0	55.0	57.2	59.6	62.2	65.0	68.1	71.5	75.3	79.5	84.1	89.4	95.4	102.1	110.0	53

Chainwheel (Front Sprocket)

Bibliography

Allen, John S. *The Complete Book of Bicycle Commuting*. Rodale Press (33 E. Minor St., Emmaus, PA 18049), 1981. Paperback: $10.95; hardcover: $14.95. Organized and written with the beginner in mind, this book describes all the skills necessary to ride confidently in traffic.

Ballantine, Richard. *Richard's Bicycle Book*. New York: Ballantine Books, 1978. Paperback: $4.95. A complete guide to buying, maintaining and repairing any bicycle. Includes exploded drawings of all complex parts.

The editors of *Bicycling* magazine. *Basic Bicycle Repair*. Rodale Press (33 E. Minor St., Emmaus, PA 18049), 1980. Paperback: $3.95. Intended for those people who want to know enough about repair to keep a bike on the road.

————. *Basic Riding Techniques*. Rodale Press (33 E. Minor St., Emmaus, PA 18049), 1979. Paperback: $3.95. Provides information on basic cycling techniques.

————. *Best Bicycle Tours; Best Bicycle Tours*, Vol. 2. Rodale Press (33 E. Minor St., Emmaus, PA 18049), 1980, 1981. Paperback: $3.95. Thirty-six tours based on the road-tested experience of *Bicycling* magazine readers.

————. *Bicycle Commuting*. Rodale Press (33 E. Minor St., Emmaus, PA 18049), 1980. Paperback: $3.95. A handbook for cyclists who want to use a bike for commuting.

————. *Get Fit with Bicycling*. Rodale Press (33 E. Minor St., Emmaus, PA 18049), 1979. Paperback: $3.95. Written by two medical doctors who give precise medical advice about general health, training schedules, nutrition, and more.

————. *The Most Frequently Asked Questions About Bicycling*. Rodale Press (33 E. Minor St., Emmaus, PA 18049), 1980. Paperback: $3.95. The most frequently asked questions about bicycling gathered into one volume for easy reference.

————. *Reconditioning the Bicycle*. Rodale Press (33 E. Minor St., Emmaus, PA 18049), 1979. Paperback: $3.95. A step-by-step guide to overhauling the bicycle.

Cuthbertson, Tom. *Anybody's Bike Book*. Ten Speed Press (900 Modoc, Berkeley, CA 94707), 1971. Paperback: $4.95. An original manual of bicycle repairs. Hand-drawn diagrams illustrate the clear step-by-step explanations.

de la Rosa, Denise M. and Michael J. Kolin. *The Ten Speed Bicycle*. Rodale Press (33 E. Minor St., Emmaus, PA 18049), 1979. Paperback: $11.95. The authors provide step-by-step instructions on how to install, adjust, and maintain every type of bicycle component.

DeLong, Fred. *DeLong's Guide to Bicycles and Bicycling*. Radnor, PA: Chilton Book Co., 1978. Paperback: $9.95. Covers touring, racing, riding to work, buying bicycles, and various aspects for enjoyable cycling.

Glenn, Harold T. and Clarence W. Coles. *Glenn's Complete Bicycle Manual*. New York: Crown Publishers

Inc., 1973. Paperback: $5.95. Comprehensive manual providing detailed step-by-step illustrated instructions for overhauling, adjusting and maintaining every part of all types of bicycles.

Johnson, Bob and Patricia Bragg, Ph.D. *The Complete Triathlon Swim, Bike and Run Distance Training Manual*. Santa Barbara, CA: Health Science, 1982. Hardcover: $24.95. A comprehensive, concise encyclopedia of multisport fitness training and covers every conceivable area of over-distance swim, bike and run training.

Kolin, Michael J. and Denise M. de la Rosa. *The Custom Bicycle*. Rodale Press (33 E. Minor St., Emmaus, PA 18049), 1979. Paperback: $10.95. This book explores the personalities, techniques, and design ideas of 20 of the world's foremost bike builders.

Lieb, Thom. *Everybody's Book of Bicycle Riding*. Rodale Press (33 E. Minor St., Emmaus, PA 18049), 1980. Paperback: $10.95; hardcover: $14.95. This helpful book thoroughly discusses planning, undertaking, and enjoying bicycle touring, from the short trip around town to the exotic excursion.

Rakowski, John. *Adventure Cycling in Europe*. Rodale Press (33 E. Minor St., Emmaus, PA 18049), 1981. Hardcover: $14.95. A practical guide to low-cost bicycle touring in 27 countries. This guidebook includes maps and narrative on terrain, language, people, and much more.

Wilhelm, Tim and Glenda. *The Bicycle Touring Book*. Rodale Press (33 E. Minor St., Emmaus, PA 18049), 1980. Paperback: $10.95; hardcover: $14.95. This helpful book thoroughly discusses planning, undertaking, and enjoying bicycle touring, from the short trip around town to the exotic excursion.

INDEX

KEEP FIT WITH WARNER BOOKS

___**HEAVYHANDS**™   (L38-004, $8.95, U.S.A.)
Leonard Schwartz, M.D.   (L38-005, $10.75, Canada)
"Heavyhands lets almost anyone move safely toward fitness . . . [This] book is more than just a workout schedule. It's a full-grown exercise system with practical and entertaining advice . . ."   *—American Health*
The newest thing in exercise.

___**RUNNING AND BEING: THE TOTAL EXPERIENCE**
Dr. George Sheehan   (L97-090, $3.95)
"George Sheehan is the first great philosopher whose body can run with his mind. **RUNNING AND BEING** examines more than the 'how to' or 'why' of running. It transcends the traditional stereotype analysis of sport and allows us to examine who we are—the runner, the man."
   —Bob Glover, co-author of *The Runner's Handbook*.

Sheehan laces his philosophy with practical advice and includes his unique one-day method for determining which sport is best for you. He tells how to prepare for a marathon, how to jog effectively, avoid injuries, and what it takes to compete in a race.
"What particularly endears George Sheehan to runners is his contagious insistence that running is something more than a sport—that it is an activity that offers glimpses of values that are profound."
   —James F. Fixx in *The Complete Book of Running*.
Available in large-size quality paperback

WARNER BOOKS
P.O. Box 690
New York, N.Y. 10019

Please send me the books I have checked. I enclose a check or money order (not cash), plus 50¢ per order and 50¢ per copy to cover postage and handling.* (Allow 4 weeks for delivery.)

_____ Please send me your free mail order catalog. (If ordering only the catalog, include a large self-addressed, stamped envelope.)

Name _____

Address _____

City _____

State _____ Zip _____

*N.Y. State and California residents add applicable sales tax.   53

IMPORTANT BOOKS
FOR YOUR BODY
FROM WARNER BOOKS

____**THE COMPLETE BOOK OF SPORTS MEDICINE**
Richard H. Dominguez, M.D.   (L37-370, $5.95)

Do you run, play tennis, basketball, football? Arm yourself against injury,
and learn what to do if you do get hurt. This book tells you:
- When to use massage, ice packs, heat, and taping in home treatment
  of an injury
- How to judge the seriousness of an injury—which ones call for a trip to
  the emergency room, which ones are "wait and see"
- Which sports are helpful, and which ones are harmful for people
  with asthma, diabetes, bad back problems
- How to prevent many common sports injuries through proper training
  and exercise

Available in large-size quality paperback

____**TOTAL BODY TRAINING**
Richard H. Dominguez, M.D., and   (L97-981, $7.95, U.S.A.)
Robert Gajda   (L37-284, $9.25, Canada)

Do you do sit-ups, deep knee bends, ballet stretches, the hurdler's stretch,
the stiff leg raise, the knee stretch? *Stop now!*—before you harm the
structure of your lower back or do injury to muscles by stressing them
beyond their normal limits. Learn how to condition yourself in a balanced
way with TOTAL BODY TRAINING. With the methods advocated by Dr.
Dominguez (orthopedic surgeon and sports physician) and Robert Gajda
(former Mr. Universe), you can develop your "core" muscles so that your
body gains the ability to withstand the stress of sudden, violent movements
that can injure you, as well as prepare yourself for the predictable strains.
Try this program of preparation and prevention that well-known sports
figures and gymnasts use, and discover the secret of sports endurance.

Available in large-size quality paperback

WARNER BOOKS
P.O. Box 690
New York, N.Y. 10019

Please send me the books I have checked. I enclose a check or money order
(not cash), plus 50¢ per order and 50¢ per copy to cover postage and handling.*
(Allow 4 weeks for delivery.)

_____ Please send me your free mail order catalog. (If ordering only the
         catalog, include a large self-addressed, stamped envelope.)

Name _____

Address _____

City _____

State _____ Zip _____

*N.Y. State and California residents add applicable sales tax.   50

THREE GREAT BOOKS FROM THE EXERCISE EXPERT, RICHARD SIMMONS

—RICHARD SIMMONS' BETTER BODY BOOK
Available in hardcover   (L51-263, $16.50 FPT)

You can redesign your body—with a little help from the pro! Richard Simmons shows you how to shape up with a slimmer, firmer, tighter body—better than it ever was before! Here is the only book that offers exercise programs for all levels of fitness, tailored to suit *you*. In these pages are over two hundred fully illustrated exercises, individually planned for a workout from head to toe. But first, you'll learn how to determine your body type, assess your level of fitness, begin at your proper exercise level, and separate truth from myth in the exercise program that can transform your body and your life!

—RICHARD SIMMONS' NEVER-SAY-DIET BOOK
                                          (L97-041, $7.95, U.S.A.)
                                          (L37-505, $9.50, Canada)

Nationally-known television star Richard Simmons gives you his volume food plan and his body-correcting exercises—a positive life-changing program geared to your individual needs. There's never been a weight-loss book like this before—informal, sensible, encouraging, filled with insights, and sound, effective ways to take off pounds and keep them off for good.

—RICHARD SIMMONS' NEVER-SAY-DIET COOKBOOK
                                          (L37-078, $7.95, U.S.A.)
                                          (L37-553, $9.50, Canada)

Phase two of Simmons' fat-fighting world plan! This companion volume to his first book presents a comprehensive program for enjoying life's culinary pleasures while staying healthy and shedding excess pounds.

WARNER BOOKS
P.O. Box 690
New York, N.Y. 10019

Please send me the books I have checked. I enclose a check or money order (not cash), plus 50¢ per order and 50¢ per copy to cover postage and handling.* (Allow 4 weeks for delivery.)

_____ Please send me your free mail order catalog. (If ordering only the catalog, include a large self-addressed, stamped envelope.)

Name _____

Address _____

City _____

State _____ Zip _____

*N.Y. State and California residents add applicable sales tax.   51

BECOME STRONGER, SHAPELIER, SEXIER!

__GETTING BUILT

Dr. Lynne Pirie with   *(L37-857, $10.95, U.S.A.)*
Bill Reynolds   *(L37-858, $13.25, Canada)*

Bodybuilding—it's more than the hottest new trend in the sports category, more than the fastest-growing sport in the world, and more than the quickest and most effective way to a beautifully toned and shaped body! For thousands of women throughout the world, bodybuilding has become *the* way to achieve the look of the eighties: sleek, muscular, graceful. This book, fully illustrated, is the complete guide for both the beginner and the advanced bodybuilder.

__FLEX APPEAL BY RACHEL

Rachel McLish with   *(L38-105, $12.50, U.S.A.)*
Bill Reynolds   *(L38-106, $13.95, Canada)*

Learn how to use bodybuilding techniques to reshape your body for long-lasting fitness and natural beauty. Whether you're a beginner or an advanced bodybuilder, you can reach your physical potential with Rachel McLish's weight training program and complete guide to sensible nutrition. Discover why bodybuilding has become the fastest growing sport in the world. You'll be on your way to becoming a better, more beautiful you!

WARNER BOOKS
P.O. Box 690
New York, N.Y. 10019

Please send me the books I have checked. I enclose a check or money order (not cash), plus 50¢ per order and 50¢ per copy to cover postage and handling.*
(Allow 4 weeks for delivery.)

_____ Please send me your free mail order catalog. (If ordering only the catalog, include a large self-addressed, stamped envelope.)

Name _____

Address _____

City _____

State _____ Zip _____

*N.Y. State and California residents add applicable sales tax.   52

Improve Your Health
with WARNER BOOKS

___**LOW SALT SECRETS FOR YOUR DIET**   *(L37-223, $3.95, U.S.A.)*
by Dr. William J. Vaughan   *(L37-358, $4.50, Canada)*

Not just for people who must restrict salt intake, but for everyone! Forty to
sixty million Americans have high blood pressure, and nearly one million
Americans die of heart disease every year. Hypertension, often called the
silent killer, can be controlled by restricting your intake of salt. This handy
pocket-size guide can tell you at a glance how much salt is hidden in more
than 2,600 brand-name and natural foods.

___**EARL MINDELL'S VITAMIN BIBLE**   *(L30-626, $3.95, U.S.A.)*
by Earl Mindell   *(L32-002, $4.95, Canada)*

Earl Mindell, a certified nutritionist and practicing pharmacist for over fifteen
years, heads his own national company specializing in vitamins. His VITA-
MIN BIBLE is the most comprehensive and complete book about vitamins
and nutrient supplements ever written. This important book reveals how
vitamin needs vary for each of us and how to determine yours; how to
substitute natural substances for tranquilizers, sleeping pills, and other
drugs; how the right vitamins can help your heart, retard aging, and improve
your sex life.

___**SUGAR BLUES**
by William Dufty   *(L30-512, $3.95)*

Like opium, morphine, and heroin, sugar is an addictive drug, yet Americans
consume it daily in every thing from cigarettes to bread. If you are overweight, or suffer from migrane, hypoglycemia or acne, the plague of the
Sugar Blues has hit you. In fact, by accepted diagnostic standards, *our
entire society is pre-diabetic. Sugar Blues* shows you how to live better
without it and includes the recipes for delicious dishes—all sugar free!

___**THE CORNER DRUGSTORE**   *large format paperback:*
by Max Leber   *(L97-989, $6.95, U.S.A.)*
   (L37-278, $8.50, Canada)

In simple, down-to-earth language, THE CORNER DRUGSTORE provides
complete coverage of the over-the-counter products and services available
at your local pharmacy. Here's everything you should know about everything that pharmacies sell, a working knowledge that will save you money
and enable you to use nonprescription drugs and health aids more wisely.

WARNER BOOKS
P.O. Box 690
New York, N.Y. 10019

Please send me the books I have checked. I enclose a check or money order
(not cash), plus 50¢ per order and 50¢ per copy to cover postage and handling.*
(Allow 4 weeks for delivery.)

_____ Please send me your free mail order catalog. (If ordering only the
catalog, include a large self-addressed, stamped envelope.)

Name _____

Address _____

City _____

State _____ Zip _____

*N.Y. State and California residents add applicable sales tax.   80

Basic Equipment for Campers, Hikers and Backpackers! from WARNER BOOKS

___**Roughing It Easy**   *(H32-489, $3.95, U.S.A.)*
by Dian Thomas   *(H32-490, $4.95, Canada)*

"It takes an outdoor woman from Utah to write a . . . complete primer on making do outdoors. It puts the commonplace into unthought-of-uses. A great cookbook."—*Phoenix Gazette*

"So filled with fantastic ideas on how to make something out of nothing that you'll be itching to go camping to try them out."—*The Albertan* (Canada)

___**Roughing It Easy #2**
by Dian Thomas   *(H30-644, $3.50)*

Enlarging on ROUGHING IT EASY's imaginative tips, this book contains selections on cooking, heating, drying, and preserving food with solar energy; hints on improvising a shower, washing machine and oven; dozens of new inviting recipes for outdoor cookery, and more than 200 diagrams, drawings and photographs!

___**BUSHCRAFT**
by Richard Graves   *(H30-890, $3.95)*

You can survive in the wilderness with only a knife and this book. It shows you how to stay alive in difficult terrain, how to find food and water, how to build a shelter, how to tell time, make traps, maps and ropes. A compendium of fascinating information about the wilds.

WARNER BOOKS
P.O. Box 690
New York, N.Y. 10019

Please send me the books I have checked. I enclose a check or money order (not cash), plus 50¢ per order and 50¢ per copy to cover postage and handling.* (Allow 4 weeks for delivery.)

_____ Please send me your free mail order catalog. (If ordering only the catalog, include a large self-addressed, stamped envelope.)

Name _____

Address _____

City _____

State _____ Zip _____

*N.Y. State and California residents add applicable sales tax.   49

Discover what cycling can do for you!

Here at last is the first complete guide to full body fitness through cycling—the remarkable sport that can trim you down, build you up, and provide life-enhancing pleasure at any age! Not since *The Complete Book of Running* has there been a manual to treat an individual sport in such comprehensive detail, including:

- How to *use your bike properly* for optimum fun and fitness
- Individualized cycling programs to help you *tone up, lose weight, lower blood pressure and cholesterol*
- What to look for and how to buy the bike that fits you best
- How to put your old bike in order
- A guide to bike touring, commuting, and recreational riding
- How to begin racing
- How to gain maximum benefits with minimum stress by using the proper pedaling technique and shifting gears
- The secret to injury-free cycling
- Basic training schedules for beginners and intermediates
- Tips from the pros
- Specialized training for long distance, hills, and more
- Staying in shape off-season: indoor and outdoor exercises
- Nutrition for cyclists
- How to use cycling as an appetite depressant
- Inspiring true stories of people who conquered physical disabilities through cycling: their regimens and secrets
- Extensive appendices, bibliography, and more

38234

0

70993 00895

ISBN 0-446-38234-5

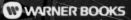

WARNER BOOKS
A Warner Communications Company

0-446-38234-5 (U.S.A.) 0-446-38235-3 (CAN.)
COVER PRINTED IN U.S.A.
© 1984 WARNER BOOKS